Anxiety in Clinical Practice

Anxiety in Clinical Practice

ANDREW SIMS AND PHILIP SNAITH
Department of Psychiatry, University of Leeds

A Wiley Medical Publication

JOHN WILEY & SONS

Chichester · New York · Brisbane · Toronto · Singapore

Copyright ©1988 by John Wiley & Sons Ltd

Distributed in the United States of America, Canada and Japan by Alan R. Liss Inc., 41 East 11th Street, New York, NY 10003, USA.

Library of Congress Cataloging-in-Publication Data
Sims, Andrew.
    Anxiety in clinical practice/Andrew Sims and Philip Snaith.
      p. cm.—(A Wiley medical publication)
    ISBN 0 471 92055 X
    1. Anxiety. I. Snaith, Philip. II. Title. III. Series.
RC531.S55 1988
616.85′223—dc19   88-17151
                                                CIP

British Library Cataloguing in Publication Data
Sims, Andrew
    Anxiety in clinical practice.
    1. Man. Neuroses: Anxiety
    I. Title II. Snaith, Philip
    616.85′223

    ISBN 0 471 92055 X

Phototypeset by Dobbie Typesetting Limited, Plymouth, Devon
Printed and bound by Biddles Limited, Guildford

Contents

Preface

Anxiety may prove to be not just a nuisance but a calamity to an individual. It can pervade every aspect of human activity and alter the way he or she sees the world to such an extent that he can no longer cope adequately with the ordinary demands of life. This can result in considerable economic cost and human suffering to the victim and his family. Anxiety added to physical disease will increase the handicap, complicate the clinical presentation so leading to much wastage of investigatory and treatment effort, and retard the healing. Anxiety may lead directly to excessive alcohol consumption with much resulting physical and social damage. Anxiety may cause failure in activities, from social and personal relationships to the passing of tests and examinations.

The detection and management of anxiety has often been a blind spot in the eye of the medical profession and their co-professionals, the clinical psychologists. Compared with depression, which has a vast literature of texts and research papers, anxiety has been the focus of little research effort. The advent of a few journals with a special focus in behavioural treatment and stress management has recently led to some correction of this imbalance but access to these may be difficult for the individual health worker who seeks to improve the quality of service to the anxious person needing help.

Traditionally doctors have responded to their patients' anxiety by prescribing drugs of a sedative type. Although these may occasionally have their uses, their dangers for abuse and potential for creating a state of dependence are widely known. Moreover they do not provide a solution to the anxiety. The alternative of psychotherapy in the past involved expensive time-consuming techniques so that it was not generally available to the vast number of anxious people requiring help. Recently, however, briefer, time-limited interventions have evolved, including self-help techniques which can be effectively carried out with little input from professional workers. It is these techniques which must now be more fully developed and applied if the problem of morbid anxiety is to be solved on a wide scale.

We were aware that no straightforward textbook existed for those who, perhaps without psychiatric or psychological training, seek to be informed of present day developments in the theory and practical management of anxiety. There are, of course, a number of books which address specific aspects of the problem, but the overall view is lacking. We have sought to provide this general survey of the topic which, avoiding technicalities, may be easily read by general medical and dental practitioners and their co-professionals, also by counsellors and others who have received no training in any of the disciplines related to medicine. We have retained our own baseline in medical practice and psychiatry, and attempted to provide sufficient guidance as to the circumstances in which it would be unwise to ignore the possibility of physical or psychiatric disorder, but it is our intention that the text may be read with profit by all who wish to be better informed to help anxious people.

ANDREW SIMS,
PHILIP SNAITH
1988

Chapter 1

Introduction: Why Worry?

This book is concerned with disturbance of function, disorder — **anxiety states** — and their treatment. However, before considering anxiety in an abnormal or pathological sense it is important to look at the normal experience and uses of anxiety. When a cautious and provident person plans for the future, a less careful person is likely to say: 'Why worry?' To which the first person may very well reply: 'I am not worried. I am just making reasonable preparations so that I won't have to worry'. This reply reveals both the qualitative and quantitative aspects of anxiety or worry.

Qualitatively, anxiety is associated with anticipation of future events; an emotion of the future occurring with threatened or anticipated loss or pain. Quantitatively, anxiety extends from the universal human activity of planning for the future — 'taking thought' — to the comprehensive and crippling state of **panic**.

In his discussion of the 'ambiguous' word anxiety, Lewis listed six characteristics:

1 It is an emotional state, with the subjectively experienced quality of fear or a closely related emotion (terror, horror, alarm, fright, trepidation, dread, scare)
2 The emotion is unpleasant
3 It is directed towards the future
4 There is either no recognizable threat or the threat is, by reasonable standards, quite out of proportion to the emotion it seemingly evokes
5 There are subjective bodily discomforts during the period of the anxiety (especially constriction of the chest)
6 There are manifest bodily disturbances

THE IMPORTANCE OF ANXIETY

Very often a person uses the experience of mild anxiety in the present prophylactically against the unpleasant emotion of more severe anxiety in the future. So anxiety becomes a spur to activity and thereby carries advantages for the survival of the individual. It becomes a stimulus for constructive activity and, if frustrated, is then increased, with further pressure for activity to cope with the adverse circumstances; this relationship is demonstrated by the Yerkes–Dodson law (Figure 1.1). There comes a time when increased anxiety does not improve performance, and it is at this stage that it is regarded as pathological.

Conceptualization of anxiety is very much based upon the ability of the subject to express his feelings, to describe them to another. This, of course, is not always possible but does not negate the presence of anxiety. Both children and mentally handicapped people without adequate verbal expression are clearly capable of experiencing anxiety of all degrees of severity, from mild apprehensiveness to panic. Although one cannot make enquiry of their subjective experience it is clear also that animals are capable of experiencing anxiety, with the customary physiological concomitants ('Dogs can learn to fear the future', W. H. Auden). This was recognized by Pavlov in observing states analogous to anxiety neurosis in his laboratory dogs following the Leningrad floods. It is also the basis for so-called **experimental neurosis** as described by Masserman. There are two main grounds for believing that animals experience anxiety: (1) they show distress with physiological evidence of arousal in circumstances that a human observer recognizes as anxiety-provoking; and (2) they are capable of anticipatory activity in response to dangerous and hence potentially anxiety-provoking situations.

Animal models of anxiety have been used extensively both for investigating the efficacy of supposed anxiolytic drugs and also for research into underlying neurological mechanisms for the occurrence of anxiety. Three main types of model in the experimental situation have been proposed: (1) that based on conflict or conditioned to fear; (2) that exploiting the uncertainty or anxiety generated by novelty; (3) that in which anxiety or aversion is chemically induced. The **conflict** tests are based on certain behaviour of the animal resulting unpredictably in either reward or punishment; the animal therefore carries out the behaviour because it is sometimes reinforced by rewards, but is apprehensive in doing so. In tests of **uncertainty** or novelty, degree of exploration in a new environment or the amount of social interaction in an unfamiliar situation is

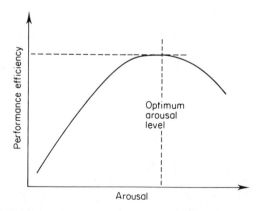

Figure 1.1: Yerkes–Dodson curve for anxiety (from Sims and Hume, 1984)

under investigation. The **chemical** induction of anxiety involves injection into an animal of a drug that is known to cause anxiety symptoms in humans, for example pentylenetetrazole. The effects of the drug upon behaviour are then ascertained and considered to be the behavioural component of anxiety in that animal. It can be seen that these model experimental situations have something in common with different aspects of human anxiety but are by no means precisely analogous.

Animal models are ultimately unsatisfactory because the phenomenology cannot be explored: that is, there can be no precise description of internal subjective experience. The human subject is capable of describing how increasing apprehensiveness and fear of anticipated loss or pain eventually results in the unpleasant emotion (or dysphoria) of anxiety. Very severe and acute anxiety is described as panic and, in the realm of psychopathology, has particular characteristics that distinguish it from less severe or more chronic experience of anxiety.

The subjective experience of anxiety in certain situations of fight and flight is a normal and necessary emotion. It both results from and further stimulates the sympathetic autonomic response to certain fear-provoking stimuli. In such situations the experience of anxiety will initially facilitate the physical response. Similarly, in some psychologically stressful situations such as making a public speech or sitting an examination a certain level of anxiety will improve performance.

The images of anxiety—its metaphors and synonyms—are in common parlance. It is well recognized as a driving force in society. Popular descriptions of being anxious concentrate upon the emotion, for example 'terrified', 'panicky', the physical concomitants—'butterflies in the stomach', 'twitchy'—and the resultant behaviour—'edgy', 'petrified'. Almost any account of an individual in a specific situation, whether it be a candidate describing how he felt in an examination or the hero in a thriller novel at a moment of high drama, will include a description of mood focused upon the parameter: terror–anxiety–apprehensiveness–tranquillity. Anxiety and its different degrees and experiences is something that people regard seriously.

A typical list of synonyms and related ideas extracted from *Roget's Thesaurus* includes amongst many others the following: **anxious**—solicitous, conscientious, scrupulous, painstaking; apprehensive, hoping, nervous, tense, keyed up, on tenterhooks.

Anxiety is accepted as a reason for behaviour, its motivation, but not as the behaviour itself. So if a person finds himself in a field with a bull, he feels anxious and as a result runs to save his life. Anxiety explains his behaviour, but running would not be thought of as anxious behaviour. However, involuntary behaviour, such as uncontrollable tremor or 'legs going weak like jelly', would be accepted as a direct manifestation of anxiety. Sometimes anxiety is used to account for behaviour when the emotion itself is not otherwise manifest, for example the so-called 'anxious searching' which occurs at an early stage following the experience of loss. This can be seen in the quiet watching of visitors to the ward by a hospitalized child after his mother has left his bedside, or alternatively following bereavement when a women may scan a street crowd to see if her dead husband is present.

The symptoms and signs of anxiety are dealt with in detail in Chapter 5. Symptoms include psychic discomfort with apprehension, fear and panic; and somatic symptoms such as muscular pains, tension headache, tremor, palpitations, diarrhoea, sweating, respiratory distress, dizziness and unsteadiness.

Normal anxiety would be regarded as an appropriate emotion to deal with particular circumstances of a situation, the emotional concomitant of the drive needed to cope with a physical or psychosocial emergency. **Abnormal** anxiety implies that the emotional response of feeling anxious and its associated behaviour either occurs without a stimulus or out of proportion to the degree of stimulus, or it persists for an unreasonable duration after the removal of the stimulus, or the consequent behaviour response is inappropriate in dealing with the threat of the stimulus.

Anxiety **state** implies a process, perhaps provoked by outside circumstances, in which the subject's normal state of equilibrium is disrupted by anxiety. **Trait** anxiety is where the development of the individual's personality results in some level of abnormal anxiety being a persistent background part of the constitution; such a person has an anxious temperament or anxiety-prone personality.

DEFINITIONS

Anxiety, then, is a necessary part of the response of the organism to external threat. However, when not provoked by a real threat, or out of proportion to the degree of danger, or persisting beyond the external stress, it has become maladaptive and constitutes **disorder**. Anxiety can be assessed according to whether the emotion is appropriate or pathological in its origin, intensity or duration. When the source of morbid anxiety is specific, it is called **phobic disorder**, and when it is generalized, **anxiety state**. **Post-traumatic stress disorder** describes the situation where anxiety with other symptoms occurs following individual catastrophe or mass disaster. Anxiety is the emotion of fearful apprehension. Cognitively, it is the emotion associated with the anticipation of an unpleasant event involving either severe discomfort, or loss, or both.

In the *International Classification of Diseases* (9th Revision, 1977), anxiety states are defined as follows: 'Various combinations of physical and mental manifestations of anxiety, not attributable to real danger and occurring either in attacks or as a persisting state. The anxiety is usually diffuse and may extend to panic. Other neurotic features such as obsessional or hysterical symptoms may be present but do not dominate the clinical picture'. This includes both anxiety and panic in the same disorder but it excludes phobic conditions.

In the classificatory system of the American Psychiatric Association (DSM IIIR, 1987), anxiety disorders are regarded as a group of conditions entirely separate from other psychiatric diagnoses. Table 1.1 lists anxiety disorders into phobic disorders, anxiety states and post-traumatic stress disorder. The rationale for

Table 1.1 Anxiety disorders in DSM IIIR

Phobic disorders (or phobic neuroses)
    Agoraphobia without panic attacks
    Social phobia
    Simple phobia
Anxiety states (or anxiety neuroses)
    Panic disorder (with or without agoraphobia)
    Generalized anxiety disorder
Post-traumatic stress disorder
    Acute
    Chronic or delayed

---

aggregating these conditions and separating them from all others is that anxiety is regarded either as the predominant disturbance as in panic disorder, or anxiety is experienced if the individual attempts to master the symptoms as in confronting the dreaded object or situation in a phobic disorder.

Both ICD 9 and DSM IIIR classifications are hierarchical in nature and a diagnosis of depression takes precedence over anxiety. This is unfortunate as a person with severe anxiety but only mild depressive symptoms, according to rigid application of the rules, should be given the diagnosis of depressive neurosis in ICD 9 or dysthymic disorder in DSM IIIR. Anxiety can, of course, cause just as much distress to the individual and disturbance in social relationships as depression. By using the statistical technique of factor analysis it has been possible to differentiate the two disorders of anxiety state and depression but they may occur at the same time in the same individual. In many patients anxiety and depressive disorders can be distinguished from each other by the constellation of symptoms experienced and the course of the illness. In some other patients there are clearly anxiety symptoms secondary to a depressive illness or alternatively depressive symptoms occurring with a predominant anxiety disorder. In other patients anxiety and depressive symptoms appear to occur together and it is impossible to decide which is the dominant condition.

Neurotic disorder, as used in ICD 9, is a useful generic category including a number of conditions which overlap, which have several features in common and which are quite different in many respects from other psychiatric disorders such as schizophrenia, dementia or manic-depressive psychosis. The anxiety disorders are found amongst neurotic disorders. In Table 1.2 are listed the separate syndromes of the neurotic disorders category in ICD 9 with their equivalent diagnosis in DSM IIIR. The authors would not accept the contention of DSM III that obsessive–compulsive disorder is an anxiety disorder, and so for the rest of this book anxiety disorder is taken to exclude obsessive–compulsive neurosis; where the latter is mentioned it is contrasted with anxiety conditions.

In the International Classification, 'neurotic disorders are mental disorders without any demonstrable organic basis in which the patient may have considerable insight and has unimpaired reality testing, in that he usually does

Table 1.2 Neurotic disorders listed in ICD 9 compared with DSM IIIR

ICD 9		DSM IIIR	
300.0	**Anxiety state**	**Anxiety state**	
		Panic disorder	300.01
		Generalized anxiety disorder	300.02
300.1	Hysteria	Somatoform disorder	
		Conversion disorder	300.11
		Dissociative disorder.	
		Psychogenic amnesia	300.12
		Psychogenic fugue	300.13
		Multiple personality	300.14
300.2	**Phobic state**	**Anxiety disorder**	
		Phobic disorders	300.2
300.3	Obsessive–compulsive disorder	Anxiety state: Obsessive–compulsive disorder	300.2
300.4	Neurotic depression	Affective disorder: Other specific affective disorder	
		Dysthymic disorder	300.40
300.5	Neurasthenia		
300.6	Depersonalization syndrome	Dissociative disorder Depersonalization disorder	300.60
300.7	Hypochondriasis	Somatoform disorder Hypochondriasis	300.70
300.8	Other neurotic disorders	Somatoform disorder Somatization disorder	300.1
		Psychogenic pain disorder	307.80
		Anxiety disorder	
		Post-traumatic stress disorder	308.30,81

not confuse his morbid subjective experiences and fantasies with external reality. Behaviour may be greatly affected although usually remaining within socially acceptable limits, but personality is not disorganized. The principal manifestations include excessive anxiety, hysterical symptoms, phobias, obsessional and compulsive symptoms, and depression'. Neurosis is a psychological reaction to acute or continuous perceived stress, expressed in emotion or behaviour ultimately inappropriate in dealing with that stress. Of course, what the patient perceives as being stressful may not necessarily be what the outside observer regards as the major source of conflict.

Neurotic conditions are inconstant in symptom and severity. They are not truly cyclical but perceived stress from either external or internal cause is likely to result in further exacerbation. Neurotic manifestations vary and one cannot predict what behaviour the neurotic person will show, nor whether symptoms will occur all the time. Neither is the nature of neurotic presentation consistent. Although phobic neurosis and depersonalization syndrome are considered separate entities, they may occur at different times in the same individual or they may occur together. The different neurotic syndromes are not mutually exclusive and a mixture of symptoms is usual rather than exceptional. Anxiety is commonly, although not universally, described in neurosis and depressive symptoms are extremely common whatever other neurotic symptoms may exist in the individual. There is a chameleon-like quality to neurotic presentation in that it tends to take on the form expected by that particular therapist or system of care: symptoms to the doctor, problems to the social worker, sins to the priest. It is important in this discussion of the symptoms of anxiety to bear in mind that these other neurotic manifestations will also be present and effective treatment of anxiety may not necessarily result in a return to normal functioning, as other symptoms may not only remain but take on increased prominence.

Concept of Stress

In any discussion of anxiety stress will necessarily be mentioned, as **anxiety** and **stress** are obverse and converse, like the faces of a coin. Whilst anxiety is a description of the subjective state, stress is the explanation by the outside observer of what he sees happening to the person who feels anxious. Stress as a factor in psychological disturbance has associations both with the mechanical concepts of stress and strain and also with the word distress, implying the metaphor of pressing too tightly and thereby causing discomfort and anguish.

The term stress is used in three quite different ways when applied to human disturbance, as shown in Figure 1.2:

1 Stress may refer to the noxious stimulus — a **stress factor**: that is, something in the external or internal environment is regarded as stressful and capable of causing a particular kind of adverse reaction, so we talk about the stress of unemployment or of examinations. Such a stress may provoke anxiety reaction either because it is intrinsically harmful or because of the particular way it is perceived by this individual person. Some external factors will therefore be construed as stresses by everyone, for instance involvement in major disaster, and others only by certain people predisposed by previous experience or by their individual constitutional and personality factors; for instance, a person lacking in self-confidence becomes acutely anxious when promoted at work.

2 Stress may refer to the nature of the response made to an external stimulus; the person responds with an experience called 'stress'. Such a person is described as being under stress and this is more a comment upon his response than on the specific nature of the external stressor. Selye considered that 'stress is the non-specific physiological response of the body to any demand made upon it'. He held stress to be a universal defensive reaction largely independent both of the type of cause and of individual variation. He considered the **general adaptation syndrome** to occur in definite stages in many different animal species. Pathological responses occurred in the so-called diseases of adaptation and the physical symptoms of anxiety were seen in this way.

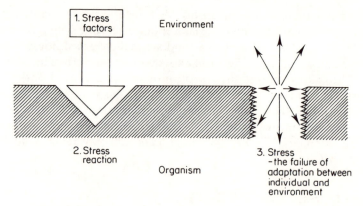

Figure 1.2: Models of stress

3 Stress may be considered to occur when there is failure of adaptation between the individual and his environment. In this, the **interactional model**, stress exists in the relationship between the person and his environment; there is a lack of fit for this individual person. This way of considering stress best accounts for the variations in biological, social and psychological state which may result in the manifestation of anxiety. So, in a variety of situations, stress is a failure of satisfactory adaptation and it becomes a system through which anxiety symptoms may be provoked by circumstances.

CLASSIFICATION

The anxiety disorders considered in this book are anxiety states (or anxiety neuroses), phobic disorders (or phobic neuroses) and post-traumatic stress disorder (or aftermath neurosis). The *International Classification of Diseases*, 9th edition, includes both generalized anxiety and panic disorder within the same condition of anxiety state. However, DSM IIIR lists three different conditions under anxiety states: panic disorder, generalized anxiety disorder, and obsessive–compulsive disorder. We have excluded the latter from further consideration. In panic disorder recurrent anxiety or panic attacks occur unpredictably though often with specific provocation, for example being in a hot, crowded lecture hall. The diagnostic criteria for the various anxiety disorders are discussed in Chapter 5.

These criteria form useful operational definitions for each condition developed for research purposes. They have the advantage of giving a relatively precise diagnosis but the disadvantage that some who are truly suffering from the condition are excluded through just failing to fulfil the criteria.

In **generalized anxiety disorder** anxiety is persistent for at least one month and is manifested in the four areas of motor tension, autonomic hyperactivity, apprehensive expectation and increased vigilance and scanning.

Panic disorder requires for diagnosis at least three panic attacks to occur in a three-week period. The attacks show such symptoms as breathlessness, palpitations, feelings of choking, sweating, and so on.

Phobic neuroses or disorders are those 'neurotic states with abnormally intense dread of certain objects or specific situations which would not normally have that effect. If the anxiety tends to spread from a specified situation or object to a wider range of circumstances, it becomes akin to or identical with anxiety state' (ICD 9). Phobias are unreasonable fears and subjectively are experienced as situational anxiety, that is, anxiety associated with specific circumstances or objects. Phobias have been classified into the categories of agoraphobia, social phobia and simple phobia.

Agoraphobia, etymologically the fear of the market place, is the occurrence of recurrent anxiety on going into a busy public place. It is frequent for sufferers to feel conspicuous and to be afraid that they will collapse and become noticeable to others. As they become increasingly concerned with this fear the somatic symptoms of anxiety increase. A prominent part of all phobic disorders is avoidance of the phobic object, so the agoraphobic housewife stops going to certain busy supermarkets; then she is unable to go into the town centre; later this extends to not being able to go out shopping on her own to the corner grocer; and finally she may become completely housebound.

Characteristic of **social phobia** is an unreasonable but persisting fear and consequent avoidance of situations in which the person may come to the notice of other people. This is associated with a fear that he or she may show behaviour that is humiliating or embarrassing. The person recognizes the unreasonableness of the fear but still cannot dispel the phobia and hence avoids the situation. In **simple phobia** there is an unreasonable and persisting fear of a specific object or situation. The commonest such fears are of animals (snakes, cats, dogs, birds, insects, and so on), but simple phobia may also be experienced for closed spaces (claustrophobia), heights (acrophobia) and for illness.

Figure 1.3 represents the different anxiety disorders diagrammatically. It needs to be borne in mind, however, that the distinction between them is often arbitrary and spurious. The different anxiety disorders merge with each other and also with other neurotic conditions. This is well evidenced for post-traumatic stress disorder, in which anxiety is often the most prominent symptom but other neurotic symptoms such as reactive depression, hypochondriasis and depersonalization are also extremely frequent; there is also overlap with the psychopathology of both phobic disorder and generalized anxiety.

The symptoms of **post-traumatic stress disorder** include reexperiencing the traumatic event and a series of stages in the emotional reaction to that event such as numbness and inertia at an early stage, and heightened anxiety and startle response which may persist for a long time, or indeed indefinitely, after the trauma has been removed. The traumatic event may be an individual circumstance such as being a victim of an assault or a participant in a road accident, or it may be a mass experience such as being involved in a natural disaster like a fire or an earthquake or a man-made catastrophe such as civilian bombing.

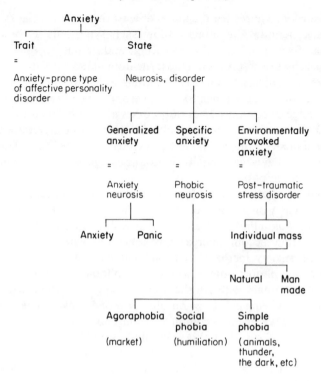

Figure 1.3: The anxiety disorders

Although the symptoms described in one individual case may point to the diagnosis of a specific anxiety syndrome, it is commoner for a mixture of anxiety and other neurotic symptoms to be present. Classification is helpful for research purposes and also for assessing what treatment methods are most likely to be successful. The different syndromes are not discrete but merge with one another.

EPIDEMIOLOGY OF ANXIETY STATES

There is no doubt that morbid anxiety is both very frequent and very disabling. Counting heads, the business of epidemiology, cannot fully do justice to the significance of this dysphoric emotion as a cause of human distress. Most people experience anxiety at some time in their lives. How commonly does it present as identifiable psychiatric disorder?

Epidemiology is the study of the distribution of diseases in different populations; in psychiatry this implies estimating the frequency of distinct types of abnormal behaviour or subjective dysphoria in defined social settings. **Prevalence** is the number of cases of a condition that is present over a specified period of time, whilst **incidence** is the number of new cases occurring in a defined period. There are difficulties with establishing the epidemiological definitions in anxiety disorders. The first problem is to decide where to make a distinction between normal anxiety with severe provocation and pathological anxiety which is regarded as illness. This concerns **caseness**, which is a major consideration for psychiatric epidemiology. An operational definition of what is a case needs to be made, for example the diagnostic criteria in Table 1.3 from the *Diagnostic and Statistical Manual* (3rd Revision — Revised) of the American Psychiatric Association (DSM IIIR) for **generalized anxiety**. The case is defined as having the required number of positive characteristics of the condition and at the same time not having other characteristics which would place the subject in a different diagnostic category.

If an abnormality is relatively infrequent in a population, like **phobia** for example, then incidence studies of the whole population will not be practicable. This would involve following a very large population over a considerable time with relatively few cases developing within the prescribed time. Prevalence studies are therefore more practicable and cost-effective. However, if a condition is of short duration, again as some phobias, then there will be a substantial difference in numbers between incidence and prevalence estimates. Of course, standardized diagnostic criteria are essential for reliable epidemiological studies and this is a reason for using a carefully described operational definition of caseness.

In order to know how common anxiety disorders are in general, surveys in the community need to be carried out rather than studies of psychiatric inpatient or hospital outpatient referrals. An earlier review of anxiety states (Weissman et al,) considered that **anxiety disorders** occurred in the lifetime of between 2.0 and 5.0 per cent of people in the general population. Weissmann, Myers and Harding (1978) reported on a large-scale community survey in which 511 randomly selected patients in New Haven, Connecticut were interviewed between 1975 and 1976 using a structured series of questions, the Schedule for Affective Disorders and Schizophrenia — lifetime version (SADS-L). Diagnosis was made according to the rules of the system called the **Research Diagnostic Criteria** (RDC). In this study the rate for all anxiety disorders was 4.3 per cent of the whole interviewed population; the subgroups of these were that panic disorder accounted for 0.4 per cent, generalized anxiety disorder for 2.5 per cent and phobic disorder for 1.4 per cent of the population.

In another study Uhlenhuth and co-workers (1983) administered a symptom checklist to more than 3000 subjects. One cannot be certain about caseness in this study; however, the one-year prevalence rate of agoraphobia with panic attacks was 1.2 per cent, of all other phobias 2.3 per cent and of general anxiety 6.4 per cent.

Anxiety disorders are commoner in women than men, the ratio usually being about 2:1. Thus for phobias, including agoraphobia, and panic disorder a ratio of 2:1 is usually given whilst generalized anxiety disorder figures of up to 3.5:1 for the female:male ratio have been given. This ratio is also maintained in those presenting for treatment, as at least twice as many women will be found in most treatment services.

Table 1.3 Diagnostic criteria for 300.02 Generalized Anxiety Disorder

A. Unrealistic or excessive anxiety and worry (apprehensive expectation) about two or more life circumstances, e.g. worry about possible misfortune to one's child (who is in no danger) and worry about finances (for no good reason), for a period of six months or longer, during which the person has been bothered more days than not by these concerns. In children and adolescents, this may take the form of anxiety and worry about academic, athletic, and social performance.

B. If another Axis I disorder is present, the focus of the anxiety and worry in A is unrelated to it, e.g. the anxiety or worry is not about having a panic attack (as in Panic Disorder), being embarrassed in public (as in Social Phobia), being contaminated (as in Obsessive Compulsive Disorder), or gaining weight (as in Anorexia Nervosa).

C. The disturbance does not occur only during the course of a Mood Disorder or a psychotic disorder.

D. At least 6 of the following 18 symptoms are often present when anxious (do not include symptoms present only during panic attacks):

Motor tension
(1) trembling, twitching, or feeling shaky
(2) muscle tension, aches, or soreness
(3) restlessness
(4) easy fatigability

Autonomic hyperactivity
(5) shortness of breath or smothering sensations
(6) palpitations or accelerated heart rate (tachycardia)
(7) sweating, or cold clammy hands
(8) dry mouth
(9) dizziness or lightheadedness
(10) nausea, diarrhoea, or other abdominal distress
(11) flushes (hot flashes) or chills
(12) frequent urination
(13) trouble swallowing or 'lump in throat'

Vigilance and scanning
(14) feeling keyed up or on edge
(15) exaggerated startle response
(16) difficulty concentrating or 'mind going blank' because of anxiety
(17) trouble falling or staying asleep
(18) irritability

E. It cannot be established that an organic factor initiated and maintained the disturbance, e.g. hyperthyroidism, caffeine intoxication.

A recent survey of the prevalence of phobias has been carried out at various sites in the USA, with lifetime prevalence varying between 7.8 per cent in New Haven and 33.3 per cent in Baltimore. Six-month prevalence from the same study, the Epidemiologic Catchment Area Study, gave six months' prevalence for social phobia 1.3 per cent for males and 1.7 per cent for females, and for simple phobia 4.3 per cent for males and 7.0 per cent for females. It is likely from the study that any error in evaluation will be an under-reporting of the true figure. For agoraphobia the lifetime prevalence ranged from 5.3 to 12.5

per cent in females and 1.5 to 5.2 per cent in males, with the six-month prevalence from 0.9 to 3.4 per cent in males and 2.7 to 5.8 per cent in females.

When the same population was used for assessment of the frequency of panic disorder, the lifetime estimates ranged from 0.6 to 1.2 per cent in males and from 1.6 to 2.1 per cent in females. The six months' prevalence ranged from 0.3 to 0.8 per cent in males and from 0.6 to 1.0 per cent in females. What is now called panic disorder probably represents the older diagnosis of **neurocirculatory asthenia**. It was estimated in 1950 that 6 per cent of patients seen in a private cardiology service were suffering from this condition.

An estimate of the prevalence of the different anxiety disorders at any particular time is shown in Figure 1.4. This has been combined from the various community studies mostly carried out in the USA (Reich, 1986). The prevalence is likely to be of the order of 3 per cent for panic disorder, 6 per cent for agoraphobia, 3 per cent for generalized anxiety, 2.5 per cent for simple phobia and 1.5 per cent for social phobia; thus at any one time about a sixth of the population will be suffering from some type of anxiety disorder, usually with a ratio of two females to one male.

It used to be considered that anxiety disorders were associated with the supposed stress of living in a developed western society. In fact, when anxiety symptoms and disorders have been looked for in different developing societies, the prevalence has been surprisingly similar to that of North America and Europe. More detailed research is required to show the precise differences between cultures.

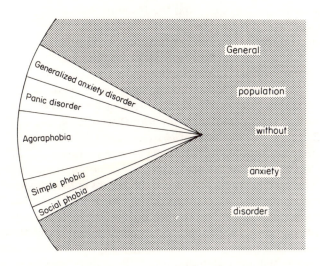

Figure 1.4: Prevalence of anxiety disorders in a general population

ANXIETY STATE—A DISEASE?

There is general agreement about the use of anxious as an adjective; usually when people feel anxious they are able to describe this and their description is accepted by other people. Anxiety as an abstract noun is somewhat more contentious and its origins are discussed in Chapter 2. However, the use of the term anxiety state is much more controversial. This implies a concept of illness, of morbidity, or of pathology. Is this justifiable?

In the next chapter an historical account is given of the transformation of anxiety from an emotion that could be a harbinger of illness to a disease entity in its own right. What is meant by the term illness or disease? **Illness** generally refers to the subjective state of the individual who feels ill and believes himself to have an illness. Very frequently it overlaps with **disease**, where objective evidence of pathology can be found.

To argue whether any particular condition of mankind should be deemed to be illness or not is fruitless. We make such distinctions on arbitrary grounds. As gardeners we want to grow potatoes and so we call potato blight a disease of potatoes. If we were more concerned to cultivate the parasite, we would regard potatoes as an ideal medium for healthy culture of the organism and select for this the variety of potato most prone to blight. So with anxiety state, if we regard it as illness, it is not because of any supposed biochemical or pathological abnormality but rather because the functioning of the individual is disturbed by it.

How do we draw the line between understandable, 'normal' anxiety and anxiety state? This is based upon the continuation of symptoms after the provoking stimulus has been removed, the severity of distress being out of proportion to the provocation, and the resultant behaviour of the individual being inappropriate to cope with the stressful situation. These three bases point to anxiety state as being essentially neurotic in nature—an adverse response to life circumstances or internal feelings or cognitions.

Sometimes anxiety that originally occurs in a specific threatening situation becomes perpetuated as a long-standing emotion of anxiety. This may occur in a **phobic state**, where there is initially fear of a particular object, situation or experience. **Avoidance** of any situation that may provoke fear leads to strengthening and prolongation of the response of anxiety.

Anxiety may be regarded as pathological because it is inappropriate in time or severity to the nature of the provocation. The notion of pathology or illness may also be invoked because of the degree of distress of the individual or because of its dire consequences—social, psychological or even physical. The World Health Organization defined health as 'a state of complete physical, mental and social well-being and not merely the absence of infirmity'. Within such a definition anxiety state is undoubtedly illness.

Using a traditional medical definition of illness being a physical disturbance, for example following Griesinger's dictum that all mental illness is disease of the brain, the case for anxiety state is more difficult to substantiate.

The evidence for a physical substrate of certain forms of anxiety state is presented in Chapter 3.

In practice most doctors regard illness as being the constellation of symptoms their patients complain of, and patients as the people who consult them requiring treatment. Despite this concept of illness being tautologous, it works well enough for most doctors in most clinical situations. Using such a definition, anxiety state is a very common illness presenting very frequently to the general practitioner; it will probably account for some presentations to medical specialists other than psychiatrists, for instance some cases of 'cardiac neurosis', 'irritable bowel', 'gritty eyes', 'stuffy nose', and so on. However, not all patients require treatment for their anxiety; and not all those requiring it will request it.

If illness is considered to convey biological disadvantage resulting in either increased mortality or decreased fecundity, then again the status of anxiety state becomes arguable. However, there is some evidence, reviewed in Chapter 4, that anxiety states are associated with increased mortality. The effects on fecundity are more difficult to demonstrate.

WHY WORRY?

The question which is the title of this chapter is deliberately ambiguous, querying both the aetiology of anxiety and why it is that particular emotion occurs in response to stimuli. The causes of anxiety from a biological and social point of view are examined in Chapters 3 and 4 respectively.

Anxiety plays an important role in the total psychological repertoire both in a normal and an abnormal state. It has been discussed that the identical emotion is regarded as an entirely appropriate response to anticipate threat and challenge in one situation and pathological in another. Anxiety may be a temporary state intervening in life or a persistent trait influencing every part of the individual's existence and behaviour. It manifests in psychological symptoms, physical complaints and also in behaviour.

Anxiety is not a unitary description but there are several discrete but overlapping anxiety disorders. Currently these are considered under generalized anxiety, phobic state, panic disorder and post-traumatic stress disorder. It is useful to consider their psychopathology separately but also to recall that these presentations often overlap and indeed commonly occur with other neurotic symptoms such as depression, irritability and sleep and other somatic disturbance.

Anxiety disorders commonly occur in the community, are very frequently complained of in primary care, and form a substantial part of the demand for psychiatric outpatient attention. Such symptoms occur in all societies where they have been studied and were frequent in the past as well as currently. Whether they should be labelled as disease depends upon definition. However, they are potent in causing distress; relief is certainly required and requested, and not inappropriately provided by mental health services.

FURTHER READING

American Psychiatric Association *Diagnostic and Statistical Manual of Mental Disorders*, 3rd edn—revised. Washington: American Psychiatric Association, 1987.

Marks, I. M. Epidemiology of anxiety. *Soc Psychiat* 1986; **21**: 167–171.

Reich, J. The epidemiology of anxiety. *J N Ment Dis* 1986; **174**: 129–136.

Sims, A. C. P. *Neurosis in Society*. Basingstoke: MacMillan, 1983.

Uhlenhuth, E. H., Balter, M. B., Mellinger, G. D. *et al.* Symptom checklist syndromes in the general population. *Arch Gen Psychiat* 1983; **40**: 1167–1173.

Weissmann, M. M., Myers, J. K. and Harding, P. S. Psychiatric disorders in a US urban community: 1975–1976. *Am J Psychiat* 1978; **135**: 459–462.

World Health Organization *International Classification of Diseases*, 9th revised edn. Geneva: WHO, 1977.

Chapter 2

Anxiety in Historical Perspective: 'That Internal Restlessness'

Although the word anxiety has only been used to describe a psychiatric syndrome during this century, the belief that this emotion of fearful apprehension could cause physical illness has a much longer history. Several early writers recognized fears, anxieties and reactions to stress as evidence of disease a long time before these conditions were fitted into nosological categories.

The earliest account of phobia is from a pupil of Hippocrates, who described two cases:

> 'Nicanor's complaint: whenever he went out drinking, dread of the flute-girl. Whenever he heard the sound of a flute beginning to play at a drinking-party, he was troubled by fears. He said he could scarcely put up with it when it was night; but if he heard it by day, he was not affected at all. Such experiences continued in his case for a long time.'

> 'Democles, the man with him, seemed to have weak sight and looseness of the body, and he said that he would not have gone by the edge of a cliff, nor on a bridge, nor would have dared to go across the shallowest of ditches, through fear that he fall, but he made his way through the ditch itself. He said that this happened to him for some time.'

Shakespeare in *The Merchant of Venice* described what may have been a phobia for cats. More comprehensive and clinically detailed descriptions of the various syndromes of anxiety disorder began in the English language with Robert Burton's *Anatomy of Melancholy* (1621).

ORIGINS OF THE WORDS: ANXIETY, PANIC AND PHOBIA

The word anxiety comes directly from the Latin *anxietas* which means troubled in mind. It is a word which has changed its meaning remarkably little over the last 2000 years; this would suggest that the internal state of human minds has not changed nearly as much as our external environment. The complex derivations of the word and its use in various European languages were traced by Sir Aubrey Lewis. He took the word back to its Indo-Germanic root *angh*, and thence *anxo* in Greek, 'to squeeze, embrace or throttle'. This became 'weighted down with grief, burdens, trouble'. Through Latin the word is traced into French, Italian and Spanish, and of course *Angst* in German, with similar original derivation, also implies narrowness and constriction (like the English word straits).

A dictionary definition of anxiety describes three uses of the word: (1) the quality or state of being anxious; uneasiness or troubled in mind about some uncertain event; solicitude, concern; (2) strained or solicitous desire; (3) (of most interest to the doctor) pathological, 'a condition of agitation and depression with a sensation of tightness and distress in the praecordial region' (*Oxford English Dictionary*). This use of the word can be traced back to 1661, when Lovell wrote about 'the Paine and Anxiety of the Ventricle'. It is, of course, also one of the classical symptoms of angina pectoris and this association has been clearly described since the middle of the last century.

The word has been used to describe a discrete emotional state since earliest times and a pathological state of anxiety has been recognized for more than three centuries to be associated with physical symptoms, especially in the chest. Difficulty in separating the meaning of the words, and therefore experience of the emotion of anxiety from depression, has also been recognized for more than a century. Psychiatrists have made a clear distinction between grief—the emotional response to the experience of loss—and anxiety—an emotional response to anticipation of harm; however, the patients they attempt to treat and try to understand are much less sure of this distinction. When Leff used a semantic differential technique, psychiatrists' concepts of anxiety and depression showed a correlation of zero— that is, they were using the words to describe two quite different emotions, whereas patients' concepts of these affects overlapped to a considerable degree.

The etymology of panic, by contrast, is much more exotic; it describes contagious emotion such as was ascribed to the influence of the god Pan. 'Sounds heard by night on mountains and in valleys were attributed to Pan and hence he was reputed to be the cause of any sudden and groundless fear' (Liddell and Scott). Although the earliest uses of the word panic implied contagion and therefore a group process, its more recent use in psychopathology has been as an individual experience of unpleasant emotion. The association with fear is significant and links panic to phobia.

The term phobia derives directly from the Greek word *phobos*, which means panic-fear or terror, and from the deity of the same name who provoked fear and panic in one's enemies. This Greek word for fear has been brought into the technical clinical vocabulary to describe intense morbid fears which are out of proportion to the apparent stimulus. Such a fear cannot be explained or reasoned away and leads to avoidance of the feared situation when possible.

Concepts in Greek Thought

The three words anxiety, phobia and panic all come down to us from Greek. From early Greek writings Onians has traced some ideas that have implications for our modern concept. The early Greeks made a distinction between *psyche*, the immortal soul, and *thymos*, the mortal mind or spirit. Psyche was associated with the head and was the immortal vitality by which a man lives. The Greeks regarded the cerebrospinal fluid as the essence of psyche and identified it with seminal fluid; thus psyche was not only a man's individual living principle, but also life transmitted in procreation. This resulted in the idea that only through chastity would a man conserve his vitality and his immortal soul. Obviously this was fertile ground for the development of anxiety and to some extent explains both mediaeval asceticism and the association between anxiety and sexuality so prominently displayed in Freud's writing.

Further developments occurred in the concept of anxiety in later Greek thinking. Hippocrates made the clinical observation that disturbed affect can result in bodily disorder. Aristotle, antedating Griesinger, concluded that every mental illness results from physical organic disease. Whilst he regarded the heart as the meeting place of all sensations, he considered that the brain had no role in sensation or perception, but was a cold, bloodless almost inorganic part of the body which absorbed the hot vapours arising from the heart. This, of course, was the origin of the later English idea of 'the vapours'; anxiety was regarded as a physical reaction. It is interesting that both phobia and panic are words describing an emotion that have in their derivation origins in a Greek god— Phobos and Pan. These gods are both the personification and were also regarded as the ultimate cause of the relevant emotion.

The Development of the Concept of Anxiety in the English Language

The characteristically English preoccupation with the individuality of things or persons really began at the time of William of Ockham in the fourteenth century. Before then, mediaeval scholasticism was much more concerned with ecclesiastical and secular roles in society, and theological issues, rather than anything pertaining to the individual person, his emotions and the precise analysis of his mental state. The effect of Ockham's theory of knowledge was to introduce a new way of looking at individuals: as important in their own right.

Any study of anxiety or depression in the English language must inevitably consider Robert Burton, whose *Anatomy of Melancholy* was published in 1621. Burton makes a distinction between the more profound states of depression (now designated psychotic) and lesser emotional disturbance such as lesser degrees of depression, anxiety and phobia. His detailed descriptions are readily recognizable by the present-day clinician. He described very accurately the agitation and anxiety that occur in profound states of depression with suicidal preoccupation and hypochondriacal delusions. For instance, psychotic intensity of anxiety is revealed in the excerpt: 'Many men are so amazed and astonished with fear that they know not where they are, what they say, what they do, and that which is worst, it tortures them many days before with continual affrights and suspicion . . . They that live in fear are never free, resolute, secure or merry but in continual pain . . .'.

Burton also describes neurotic disorders: 'Montanus speaks of one that durst not walk alone from home for fear that he should swoon or die. A second fears every man he meets will rob him, quarrel with him or kill him. A third dares not venture to walk alone, for fear he should meet the Devil; a thief; be sick: fears all old women as witches; and every black dog or cat he sees he suspecteth to be a Devil; every person comes near him is malificiated; every creature, all intend to hurt him, seek his ruine; another dares not go over a bridge, come near a pool, rock, steep hill, lye in chamber where cross beams are for fear he be tempted to hang, drown or precipitate himself. If he be in a silent auditory, as at a sermon, he is afraid he shall speak aloud, at unawares, something undecent, unfit to be said. If he be locked in a close room, he is afraid of being stifled for want of air, and still carries bisket, aquavitae, or some strong waters about him, for fear of deliquiums, or being sick; or if he be in a throng, middle of a church, multitude, where he may not well get out, though he sit at ease he is certase affected. He will freely promise, undertake any business beforehand; but when it comes to be performed he dares not adventure, but fears an infinite number of dangers, disasters, etc. . . . They are afraid of some loss, danger, that they shall surely lose their lives, goods, and all they have; but why they know not'.

The concept of **nerves** was introduced in 1667 by Willis, who considered the cause of hysteria not to be in the womb, but in 'the brain and the nervous stock'. At about this time, Richard Flecknoe described a patient with anxiety state as 'one who troubles herself with everything'.

James Vere, who was not a doctor but a merchant and a governor of Bethlem Hospital, wrote a book in 1778 entitled *A Physical and Moral Enquiry into the Causes of that Internal Restlessness and Disorder in Any Man Which has been the Complaint of All Ages*. This forerunner of Freud by 150 years ascribed anxiety to an 'internal war' between the 'lower order of instinct' and the 'moral instincts': 'It has been observed, that the lower order of instincts, which are common in other animals are exerted chiefly, if not wholely, in the preservation and continuation of their existence. But the intellectual moral instincts have a much more extensive power and influence. And although they co-operate with those, which are annexed to animal life for all good purposes of self-preservation; yet wherever that partiality or self-love prevails which is inherent in every individual and often carries a man to trespass upon that good order which Providence has established; there these intellectual, moral instincts, are often found to interpose; and from their immutable attachment to truth and equity are so far from uniting with those seducing affections, that they fail not to oppose every act of immorality; and carry with them an evidence of regret, reproach; thus creating a sort of internal war which divides a man against himself, and hence a large share of disquiet and restlessness with the unavoidable consequence'.

The first description of *unconscious motivation* ruling action has been ascribed to Theophrastus Bombastus von Hohenheim, known as Paracelsus. In 1702, Stahl generated the theory of the unconscious origin of symptoms resulting from instinctual drives becoming repressed. Francis Hutcheson, 1728, Professor of Moral Philosophy in Glasgow, was interested in the workings of the mind, considering that feelings were 'not so much in our Power, as some seem to imagine'. He made a commonsense plea to understand emotions by making enquiry of the subject: 'We saw how impossible it is for one to judge of the degree of happiness or misery in others, unless he knows their opinions, their Associations of Ideas, and the Degree of their Desires and Aversions'. Another philosopher, Jeremy Bentham, was concerned with the **psychodynamics**. He stressed the importance of 'springs of action' and 'motives' and introduced the term 'psychological dynamics'. He showed that many of our 'actual desires and motives' are unacceptable to ourselves and have to be disguised and clothed respectably by being 'ascribed to another . . . motive' by a 'sort of fig leaves'.

Behavioural theories for the onset of anxiety symptoms and also for their treatment have always existed, even though the theory of **behaviourism** is much more recent. For example, Jeremy Taylor in 1660 describes anxious fears associated with obsessional ideas: 'The scrupulous man is timorous and sad, and uneasy, and knows not why . . . Scruple is a little stone in the foot, if you set it upon the ground it hurts you, if you hold it up you cannot go forward; it is a trouble where the trouble is over, a doubt when doubts are resolved . . . we must rudely throw it away'. This latter advice, **thought-stopping**, is helpful in that it does describe what has to be achieved but unhelpful in that it does not tell the patient how he should do this. The intellectual roots of what later became known as behaviourism lie in the writings of James Mill, the father of John Stewart Mill. James Mill was an uncompromising associationist who stated: 'Ideas spring up or exist in the order in which the sensations existed, of which they are the copies'.

The differentiation of different types of personality has been made for a long time: that is, it was noted that personality is consistent through life, manifests itself in relatively fixed patterns of behaviour and is associated to some extent with physical constitution. This was expounded in the Greek (and also Ayurvedic) theory of humours linking personality and physical constitution, in that temperaments such as **sanguine** or **choleric** were considered to be linked to preponderance of that particular body fluid, blood or bile, affecting the whole body. It was recognized that temperament was closely associated with behaviour. A typical eighteenth-century example of this is shown in Figure 2.1, which is taken from a tombstone in Dorchester Abbey. This ascribes as cause of death 'excessive sensibility', anxiety and misery presumably superimposed upon personality of sensitive type — 'too delicately spun to bear the rude shakes and jostlings which we meet with in this transitory world'. Anxiety has long been known to be conducive towards psychological distress and its consequent behaviour.

Before discussing the specific words used to describe different varieties of the expression of 'anxiety', we should mention the influence of the Dane, Søren Kierkegaard, on the development of the concept. In *The Concept of Dread* (1844) he wrote: '. . . he who has observed the contemporary generation will surely

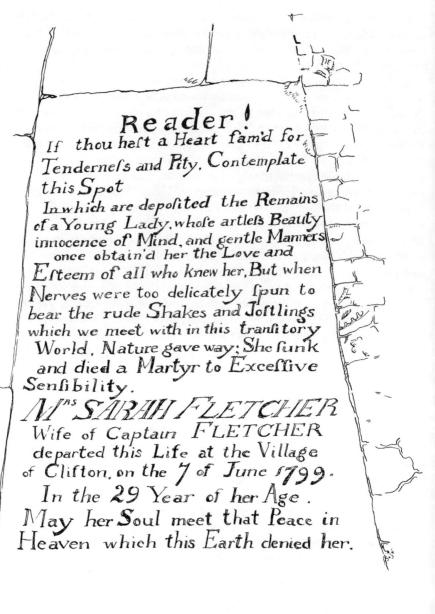

Reader!
If thou heft a Heart fam'd for
Tendernefs and Pity, Contemplate
this Spot
In which are depofited the Remains
of a Young Lady, whofe artlefs Beauty
innocence of Mind, and gentle Manners
once obtain'd her the Love and
Efteem of all who knew her, But when
Nerves were too delicately fpun to
bear the rude Shakes and Joftlings
which we meet with in this tranfitory
World, Nature gave way: She funk
and died a Martyr to Exceffive
Senfibility.
Mrs SARAH FLETCHER
Wife of Captain FLETCHER
departed this Life at the Village
of Clifton, on the 7 of June 1799.
In the 29 Year of her Age.
May her Soul meet that Peace in
Heaven which this Earth denied her.

Figure 2.1: Inscription on an eighteenth century tombstone in Dorchester Abbey

not deny that the incongruity in it and the reason for its anxiety and restlessness
is this, that in one direction truth increases in extent, in mass, partly also in
abstract clarity, whereas certitude steadily decreases'. This existential 'fear of
nothingness' was echoed in Auden's *The Age of Anxiety* one hundred years
later, the age he refers to being a time of war, the threat of ultimate annihilation.

May (1950) has summarized this: '. . . in philosophical terms anxiety arises as the individual is aware of being as over against the ever present possibility of non-being'.

THE DELINEATION OF SYNDROMES

Phobia

Pathological fears, or phobias, were described first by Hippocrates and later, in graphic detail, by Robert Burton. Benjamin Rush (1798) defined phobia as 'a fear of an imaginary evil, or an undue fear of a real one'; he then produced a list of 18 phobias, partly humorously intended, which is reproduced in Table 2.1. Agoraphobia, fear of the market place, was originally described by Westphal as a psychiatric syndrome in 1871. When he introduced the term, the three male patients whom he described demonstrated: 'impossibility of walking through certain streets or squares, or the possibility of doing so only with resulting dread of anxiety . . . agony was much increased at those hours when the particular streets were deserted and the shops closed. The patients derived great comfort from the companionship of men or even an inanimate object such as a vehicle or cane. The use of beer or wine also allowed the patient to pass through the feared locality with comparative comfort. One man even sought, without immoral motives, the companionship of a prostitute as far as his own door'.

In 1879 Maudsley quoted Westphal's description and designated phobic disorder as a separate syndrome; however, by 1895 he had included it under the general heading of melancholia. In this year also Freud distinguished between fears that were common to all mankind and specific circumstances which do not normally instil fear, for example agoraphobia. Kraepelin, in 1918, described irrepressible ideas and irresistible fears, that is, obsessions and phobias.

Anxiety State

The earliest descriptions of what later came to be recognized as anxiety neurosis ascribed the condition to a cardiac rather than a neurotic origin, thus Da Costa

Table 2.1   Species of Phobia according to Rush (1798)

1. The Cat Phobia	10. The Faction Phobia
2. The Rat Phobia	11. The Want Phobia
3. The Insect Phobia	12. The Doctor Phobia
4. The Odour Phobia	13. The Blood Phobia
5. The Dirt Phobia	14. The Thunder Phobia
6. The Rum Phobia	15. The Home Phobia
7. The Water Phobia	16. The Church Phobia
8. The Solo Phobia	17. The Ghost Phobia
9. The Power Phobia	18. The Death Phobia

(1871) described 'soldier's heart', with classical anxiety symptoms. This of course relates back to earlier work connecting anxiety with its resultant physical sensations of constriction in the praecordial region and supposed disorder of the heart.

The first paper describing anxiety neurosis as a separate syndrome was written by Hecker in 1894. In 1895, Freud's paper 'On the grounds for detaching a particular syndrome from neurasthenia under the description of "anxiety neurosis"' was published. In this paper he not only describes the psychological symptoms of anxiety neurosis but also the physical experience of panic attacks: 'An anxiety attack may consist of a feeling of anxiety alone, without any associated ideas, or accompanied by the interpretation that is nearest to hand such as ideas of the extinction of life, or a stroke, or the threat of madness . . . or the feeling of anxiety may have linked to a disturbance of one or more of the bodily functions — such as respiration, heart action, vaso-motor innervation or glandular activity. From this combination the patient picks out in particular now one, now another, factor. He complains of "spasms of the heart", "difficulty in breathing", "outbreaks of sweating" . . . and such like; and in his description, the feeling of anxiety often recedes into the background'. This was the seminal paper which established anxiety state as a separate condition.

An interesting observation on the social and occupational causation of anxiety is provided by Charles Thackrah (Figure 2.2), a medical practitioner responsible for the care of poor patients in the slums of Leeds and a founder of the Leeds Medical School in 1831. He considered that the health of doctors was particularly likely to be impaired by 'anxiety of mind'. 'Our office requires that a considerable portion of time be daily devoted to study, and the rest to professional visits. These, of course, afford exercise in the open air and thus tend to invigorate health; while on the contrary the application of mind to research tends to impair it . . . anxiety of mind does more to impair health, than breach of sleep, nocturnal exposure, or irregularity in meals. The body suffers from the mind. That sense of responsibility which every conscientious practitioner must feel, — the anxious zeal, which makes him throw his mind and feelings to cases of a special danger or difficulty, — break down the frame, change the face of hilarity to that of seriousness and care, and bring on premature age.'

Physical explanations of the causation of the disease entity of anxiety state could be considered to start in the mid-nineteenth century with, for example, Wilhelm Griesinger formulating the notion that psychological reactions are due to underlying reflex actions of the brain; anxiety thus becomes an epiphenomenon of disturbance in brain functioning. Pavlov observed the acute anxiety provoked in his dogs by the Leningrad flood and used the explanation of the occurrence of a **conditioned reflex** to account for the development of persistent anxiety whenever the dogs were exposed to similar experimental conditions of flooding. This was followed by much work on experimental neurosis carried out on animal behaviour in the 1920s. Pavlov considered that anxiety neurosis was characterized by excessive excitation with an associated loss of inhibitory processes.

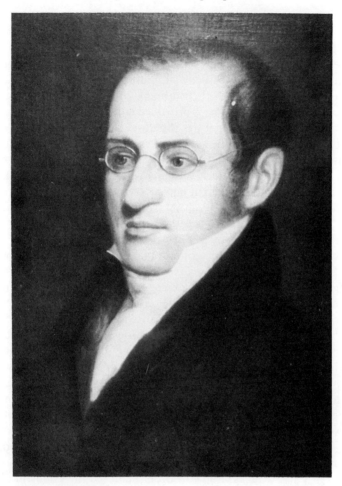

Figure 2.2: Charles Thackrah

Modelling human anxiety upon experimental neurosis in animals was further developed by Masserman. He considered that four **biodynamic** principles guide behaviour: (1) all behaviour is fundamentally motivated by the physiological requirements of the organism; (2) behaviour is adaptive; (3) behaviour is symbolic; (4) when physical inadequacies, environmental stresses or motivational conflicts exceed an organism's capacities for adaptation, then behaviour becomes hesitant, inefficient, inappropriate or excessively symbolic—that is, neurotic.

Panic Disorder

Organic and physiological explanations of anxiety have been important also in the development of the modern concept of panic disorder. However, before tracing this further we should consider again Freud's concept of panic. This he developed in a paper in 1920 entitled 'Two artificial groups: the Church and the Army'. In this paper Freud's views are expressed: 'It is not to be expected that the usage of the word "panic" should be clearly and unambiguously determined. Sometimes it is used to describe any collective fear, sometimes even fear in an individual when it exceeds all bounds, and often the name seems to be reserved for cases in which the outbreak of fear is not warranted by the occasion . . . Fear in an individual is provoked either by the greatness of a danger or by the cessation of emotional ties (libidinal cathexes); the latter is the case of neurotic fear or anxiety. In just the same way panic arises either owing to an increase of the common danger or owing to the disappearance of emotional ties which holds the group together; the latter case is analogous to that of neurotic anxiety'. This paper emphasizes that panic is a collective emotion communicated by others in a state of fear and resulting from the breakdown of a social group that may occur, for example, when the general is killed in battle.

In Freud's earlier paper on anxiety neurosis, he expresses the view quite clearly that panic attacks are related to agoraphobia: 'In the case of agoraphobia . . . we often find the recollection of an anxiety attack; and what the patient actually fears is the occurrence of such an attack under the special conditions from which he believes he cannot escape it'. Thus Freud recognizes the interconnections between the three presentations of generalized anxiety, phobia and panic.

It is only much more recently that panic disorder has been considered a distinct nosological entity. Pitts and McClure in 1967 demonstrated that sodium lactate infusion into patients with a history of spontaneous panic attacks will induce such an attack whereas its infusion into normal subjects would not. Thus a chemical means was used to induce a psychiatric symptom. Further pharmacological evidence came from the finding that tricyclic drugs and monoamine oxidase inhibitors blocked the occurrence of panic attacks in those who were otherwise prone to them, even in the absence of any overt depression. Benzodiazepines were found to be effective for generalized anxiety but did not prevent the occurrence of panic attacks. Panic disorder achieved the doubtful distinction of disease status only in 1980 in the *Diagnostic Manual* (3rd Revision) of the American Psychiatric Association; this was largely based on the above physiological and pharmacological evidence. This modern usage of the term panic disorder has not taken into account the earlier associations of the word panic with collective dysphoria.

THE AGE OF ANXIETY

Such terms as anxiety state, anxiety neurosis, anxiety reaction, phobic disorder and panic disorder are twentieth-century ideas. This is partly the legacy of Freud and other medical writers of the late nineteenth century; it could also be because we are now more aware of and better able to treat the anxiety that has always been present in individuals in society; or it could be that twentieth-century societies, especially those that are totalitarian, have induced anxiety states on a larger scale and to a greater extent within a defined population than ever previously. Post-traumatic stress disorder, some synonyms and near synonyms of which are shown in Table 2.2, involves psychological damage resulting in neurotic conditions such as chronic anxiety state; it is particularly likely to occur amongst persecuted people undergoing severe man-made trauma. Amongst such people anxiety may be induced with extreme stress in those who showed no clinically manifest signs of social maladjustment or abnormality of personality before the assaults on their psychological equilibrium.

The twentieth century has also been characterized by the popularization of Freud's emphasis of sexuality as an influence throughout life experience; thus Freud considered that when sexual tension leading to sexual desire was checked and could not be expressed, the tension was transformed into anxiety. The state of anxiety and its physical concomitants were reckoned to be somatic in their nature and not susceptible of psychological analysis. He regarded anxiety neurosis as the somatic counterpart of hysteria, in that anxiety was evoked by somatic sexual excitation whilst hysteria was caused by psychical conflict.

Medical and psychopathological use of such terms as anxiety state and anxiety neurosis was established by the 1920s. For example, Ross in *The Common Neuroses* defined anxiety reaction as 'a series of symptoms, which arises from faulty adaptation to the strains and stresses of life. It is caused by over-action in the attempt to meet the difficulties. The symptoms are those of the positive emotional reaction. They may occur in any region of the body. They may be regarded as representing an ineffectual struggle against a difficult environment'. Adler described in *Individual Psychology* the way 'that a child will make use of anxiety in order to arrive at its goal of superiority—of control over the mother'.

The earliest follow-up study of neurosis (and therefore of prognosis) also dates back to 1925. Grant followed up 665 men diagnosed as **effort syndrome** whilst they had served in the British Army during the First World War. Follow-up was five years later and 90.4 per cent were traced. At this time cardiac disease was still inextricably associated with anxiety state, although Grant considered cardiac disease not to be the underlying cause of effort syndrome. During the Fist World War there was much attention given to the related conditions of effort

Table 2.2   Some terms used for neurosis following an environmental precipitant

Post-traumatic stress disorder	
Accident neurosis	Justice neurosis
Traumatic neurosis	Triggered neurosis
Fright neurosis	American disease
Traumatic hysteria	Mediterranean disease
Traumatic neurasthenia	Greek disease
Compensation neurosis	Wharfies back
Compensationitis	Railway spine
Profit neurosis	Aftermath neurosis
Litigation neurosis	Disability neurosis
Unconscious malingering	Non-organic post-accident syndrome

syndrome, shellshock and battle neurosis. However, it was not until extensive psychiatric interest in the Second World War that the association of these with anxiety state was fully demonstrated. Much of the work that has subsequently been developed in the concept of post-traumatic stress disorder was initiated by detailed study of the victims of Hiroshima, the *hibakusha*. It was shown that irrespective of any physical damage there was very severe psychological trauma experienced by those who were involved, and this could be long-lasting if not permanent. Such severe and long-lasting psychological trauma has also been observed in those who experience other forms of trauma such as the survivors of German concentration camps or prisoners-of-war in Japanese hands during the Second World War. Symptoms of both anxiety and depression occur.

'HYSTERIC JULAP', 'PUTTING IN A PLEASED CONDITION', AND OTHER REMEDIES

When **organic** theories of aetiology have predominated, this has logically resulted in physical, and especially chemical, methods of treatment; **psychological** theories of aetiology have given rise to what used to be called **moral** methods of treatment, and more recently have separated into psychodynamic, behavioural, cognitive and social forms of management.

In the early associations of anxiety with disease it was regarded as a symptom of cardiac illness and so the recommended treatment was organic. Thus, Lovell, in his section on 'The pain and anxiety of the ventricle', recommends 'narcotics and anodynes if need, mucilages, things fat and emplastick, emulsions and roborants' for its treatment. Similarly Thomas Sydenham, writing 20 years later, recommended in the treatment of what he designated hysterical disorders, which are very close to our modern concept of neuroses, 'bleeding, purging, opiates, foetid medicines, chalybeate medicine, filings of steel and rhenish wines, plaister at the navel, hysteric julap, opening pills or electuary', and many other dramatic, physical remedies. The more specific use of psychopharmacology for the treatment of anxiety state was described by Sir Richard Blackmore, physician to Queen Anne, who explained why he used opium for this condition: 'it calms and soothes the Disorders and Perturbations of the animal Spirits; which when lulled and charmed by this soporiferous drug cease their Tumults and settle into a State of Tranquility: wonderful it is, how soon the Hurry and Tempest in the Nerves is composed by the Solicitation and Intervention of this prevailing Medicine' — a fulsome panegyric unequalled by the advertisements of the modern pharmaceutical industry.

It was well recognized, however, that drugs and other physical methods of treatment were not effective in all cases. James Howell, for instance, made the important point: 'It is true that ther may be som distempers of the mind that proceed from those of the body, and so are curable by drugs and diets; but ther are others that are quite abstracted from all corporeal impressions, and are merely mental; these kind of agonies are the more violent of the two . . .'. This non-pharmacological treatment of anxiety was characterized by Richard

Baxter, a seventeenth-century minister, the essence of whose treatment was to 'put them in a Pleased condition'; this was the opposite of so much current medical practice which consisted in administering discomfort, pain and shock. Downame, another Puritan clergyman, recommended the use of silence in his book *Spiritual Physicke to Cure the Diseases of the Soul*, which amounted to an early text of psychotherapy.

Moral methods of treatment in psychiatry included what would now be regarded as the principles of the therapeutic milieu and also individual psychotherapy; attention was paid to the therapeutic atmosphere of psychiatric wards towards the end of the eighteenth century especially by William Tuke, Phillipe Pinel, and others. The term psychotherapy was introduced into England in 1853 by Dendy in his paper 'psychotherapeia for the remedial influences of mind'. The introduction of the principles of group psychotherapy can be ascribed to Samuel Tuke in his 'Practical hints concerning the building of Wakefield asylum'.

The development of more effective methods of treatment of anxiety with psychopharmacology, abreactive techniques, behavioural modification and anxiety management methods are of course much more recent in origin. Barbiturates were extensively used for the treatment of anxiety but their dangers are well known and the introduction of the benzodiazepines resulted in barbiturates becoming obsolete in this context. Systematic desensitization as a treatment for anxiety was reported by Wolpe in 1958, whilst Autogenic Training had been introduced by Schultz, who introduced it in the 1920s as a method of treatment for anxiety.

SUMMARY

Anxiety is an old word that has changed surprisingly little in meaning since its classical origins. Both phobia and panic took their origins as the personification of emotion in Greek gods. Anxiety was used in medicine in the seventeenth century, with somatic concomitants always an essential part of the symptomatology; the link with cardiac disease has been particularly close. Use of the word in psychiatry occurred in the nineteenth century as **agitation** in depressive psychosis, but not really until the 1920s as **anxiety neurosis**. Phobias associated with disordered mental states have been described since Hippocrates but agoraphobia as a separate syndrome was delineated in the mid-nineteenth century; since then the condition has been categorized and defined. Although panic was described by Freud at the end of the nineteenth century, panic disorder has only been categorized since 1980.

Anxiety neurosis has been seen as one form of neurotic disorder; it is not entirely distinct from other types of neurotic disability such as phobic neurosis or depressive neurosis. Anxiety as one of the symptoms occurring without organic cause, has always been common as a presentation amongst the patients a doctor sees. Doctors have quite often regarded anxiety as evidence of organic disease; sometimes recognized there to be no physical basis for this symptom; more rarely, they have realized also that there are psychological explanations for it. Anxiety has always been the symptom at the boundary between physical disturbance and disorder of mind; it is experienced both somatically and psychologically, and it is also caused both by physical illness and emotional conflict.

As for other neurotic conditions, organic and psychological theories for both aetiology and treatment have run in parallel; as sedative drugs have been discovered and introduced into the pharmacopoeia, they have been used for the treatment of anxiety. Similarly, different types of psychotherapeutic approach have been used with variable success. The word anxiety, that was used either in a non-medical setting or linked with known organic disease in previous centuries, has in this century, through the work of Freud, Pavlov and others, become used in psychiatry, not only as the description of a symptom but also the name of the supposed disease.

FURTHER READING

Auden, W. H. *The Age of Anxiety*. London: Faber & Faber, 1948.

Freud, S. On the grounds for detaching a particular syndrome from neurasthenia under the description 'anxiety neurosis'. *Standard Edition of the Complete Psychological Works of Sigmund Freud*, Vol. III, pp. 90–115. London: Hogarth Press, 1895.

Hippocrates. Epidemics V, Sec. 81, 82; VII, Sec. 86, 87. In Littre, E. *Oeuvres Complètes d'Hippocrate*, Vol. 5. Paris: Baillière, 1846. (Trans. from Greek, Smart, J. 1988).

Lewis, A. Problems presented by the ambiguous word 'anxiety' as used in psychopathology. In *Later Papers of Sir Aubrey Lewis*. Oxford: Oxford University Press, 1977.

May, R. *The Meaning of Anxiety*. New York: Ronald Press, 1950.

Sims, A. C. P. Historical aspects of anxiety. *Postgrad Med J* 1988; **64**(Suppl. 2), 3–9.

Chapter 3

The Biological Basis
of Anxiety

Anxiety is traditionally conceptualized as an understandable response to stress by an individual primed by prior experience to respond in this way. However, all psychic events have a neural substrate and the demonstration of a biological basis for some mental disorders leads to increasing interest in the neuro-pathological aspects of anxiety. Prior experience alone accounts inadequately for the observation that of two similar individuals exposed to the same stress, one may rapidly regain poise whilst the other is prone to a pervasive and an enduring state of fear. Personality traits including proneness to anxiety, 'neuroticism' and shyness have been studied and there is some evidence of a predisposition, independent of experience, for the individual to be anxious. The recent focus of attention on a type of anxiety state termed panic disorder and its response to pharmacological treatment has led to a quickening of interest in the biological investigation of anxiety disorder.

GENETIC STUDIES

It has repeatedly been shown that anxiety is familial and that parents and children or brothers and sisters have similar degrees of proneness to anxiety or develop similar anxiety states. However, these observations may be entirely accounted for by imitation and learning and they provide no evidence for an inherited predisposition to anxiety. Twin studies provide an opportunity to observe the relative contributions of heredity and environment, for identical or monozygotic (MZ) twins have identical genetic endowment whereas dizygotic (DZ) twins are not more similar in their genetic endowment than ordinary siblings. Even in twin studies it is probable that similarity in the pattern of rearing and the closer identification of MZ twins with each other will play a part in the development of traits; only the critical study of twins separated at birth and reared in different environments can provide confident evidence for genetic endowment of psychological disorders. In the area of anxiety no such studies have been under-taken. Another major impediment is that anxiety states are not a homogeneous condition and some forms precede or follow the appearance of other psychiatric disorders, such as affective disorder, in which the genetic basis is more firmly established. Nevertheless a very much higher concordance of anxiety in MZ than in DZ twins is a pointer towards a hereditary and biological basis.

There have only been two such studies. In 1971 Slater and Cowie reported seven out of 17 MZ twins (41 per cent) and one out of 28 DZ twins (4 per cent) concordant for anxiety disorder. A larger series with a more careful analysis of the type of anxiety disorder was reported by Torgersen in 1983. The study covered the whole of the country of Norway and all patients reporting to a psychiatric insitution, either as an inpatient or an outpatient within a defined age range and time period, were studied. The anxiety disorders were diagnosed, using the DSM III system, into panic disorder, agoraphobia with and without panic, social phobia, obsessive–compulsive disorder and generalized anxiety disorder; 85 twin pairs were identified. For generalized anxiety disorder there was no difference in concordance between MZ and DZ twins; for the panic disorder and the agoraphobia with panic groups combined, two of 13 MZ twins and none of 16 DZ twins were concordant which provides weak evidence for a genetic basis. Even for the panic disorder syndrome, which is thought most likely to have a biological basis, the MZ concordance is far below 100 per cent, indicating that environmental factors are the prime determinant.

NEUROANATOMICAL SYSTEMS

The historical development of ideas concerning the somatic basis of emotions and particularly of anxiety can be traced. In the seventeenth century the philosopher Descartes proposed that the body and the mind functioned in parallel but did not interact; thus bodily sensations could be perceived and emotional states experienced, but the one did not influence the other. This so-called dualist theory held sway until the nineteenth century when an American psychologist, William James, and a Danish anatomist, C. Lange, independently proposed that emotional experience is based upon the perception of bodily sensations: thus a startling experience causes the heart to beat rapidly and the awareness of this physiological state gives rise to the emotion of anxiety. According to James:

> 'Common sense says we lost our fortune, are sorry and weep; we meet a bear, are frightened and run; we are insulted by a rival, are angry and strike. The hypothesis here to be defended says that this order of sequence is incorrect, that the one mental state is not unduly influenced by the other, that the bodily manifestations must first be interposed between, and that the more rational statement is that we feel sorry because we cry, angry because we strike, afraid because we tremble.' (Quoted by Tyrer, 1976)

This view was dubbed the James–Lange hypothesis of emotion.

In 1915 W. B. Cannon published his observations in a book *Bodily Changes in Pain, Hunger, Fear and Rage*. Cannon considered the emotional experience to be primary and the bodily changes to be the consequence—a reversal of the James–Lange view. Among the physiological responses to emotional situations, he defined the 'fight or flight' reaction whereby the body prepares itself to deal with threat. In this response to threat, a major role is subserved by the activity of the autonomic nervous system and especially the β-adrenergic fibres of the sympathetic division of the system. The blood supply to the skin diminishes— 'going pale with fear'—and this, together with the increase in heart rate and suspension of digestive processes, diverts blood to supply the musculature, the pupils of the eyes dilate promoting visual acuity and sweating may occur in order to keep the body cool. In 1927 Cannon proposed his 'alternative explanation' to the James–Lange theory; he considered that the thalamus was the information clearing house for emotional expression, connecting through its afferent and efferent fibres to the cerebral cortex and to the autonomic nervous system.

In 1937 Papez proposed that parts of the brain phylogenetically subserving the sense of smell are elaborated in man to subserve emotional expression. Papez's 'circuit' comprises the mamillary bodies, the fornix, anterior thalamic nuclei, the parahippocampal and the cingulate gyri; from these structures there are close neuronal connections with the temporal lobes. The relation of the latter structures to emotion is underlined by the rich and varied disorders of emotional expression which occur in disorder of temporal lobe function and especially temporal lobe epilepsy.

Gray (1981), basing his reasoning on the behavioural effects of benzodiazepine drugs, has studied the emotional basis of anxiety and has highlighted the importance of the septohippocampal system. This area of the brain receives information and compares 'actual' with 'expected' experience. This is the basis

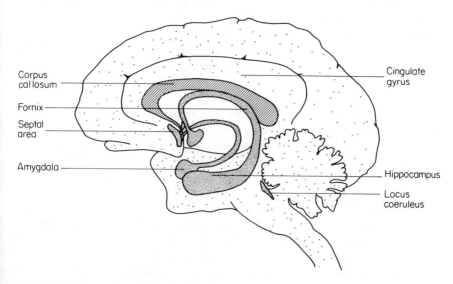

Figure 3.1: Section through the brain showing the position of structures mentioned in the text

of vigilance; when the stimulus is 'expected', ongoing activity is not interrupted and the animal may continue to browse or to execute learned behaviour but as soon as there is a mismatch, i.e. the actual fails to match the expected perception, then ongoing activity is interrupted and the animal prepares for action by increased alertness and alternative behavioural strategies, like fleeing or investigation, are instituted. Important classes of 'mismatch' events include novelty, threat and omission of expected reward. The septohippocampal system has links with the pathways identified by Papez as being the basic substrate of emotional experience; there are also important connections with a structure at the floor of the fourth ventricle called, from its bluish colouration, the locus coeruleus. Descending pathways from the locus coeruleus affect the sympathetic nervous system and this cluster of cells has therefore a key role in the transmission of neuronal information subserving the experience of anxiety.

A study using positron emission tomography (PET) was conducted in 1984 by Reiman and his colleagues. Seven patients with a history of panic attacks precipitated by sodium lactate infusion were compared with non-panic patients and found to have a significant abnormal asymmetry of cerebral blood flow in a region of the parahippocampal gyrus. The authors partly replicated their findings on a further sample but the importance of the study awaits further evaluation.

Figure 3.1 shows the position of structures in the brain referred to above.

NEUROTRANSMITTER FUNCTIONS

The transmission of neuronal information within the nervous system depends upon certain chemical systems which facilitate the passage of nervous impulses along the neurons and across the synaptic junctions from one neuron to the next in the chain. The two neurotransmitter systems most widely studied because they subserve nervous function in the neuronal substrate of mood disorder are the indoleamine (tryptophan → 5-hydroxytryptamine (serotonin) → 5-hydroxyindole acetic acid) and catecholamine (tyrosine → dopamine → noradrenaline → vanillyl mandelic acid) systems. These are important to an understanding of the mode of action of antidepressant drugs in anxiety as well as depression. The major inhibitory neurotransmitter substance is γ-aminobutyric acid or GABA. For those neuronal systems which depend upon GABA-ergic transmission there are receptors in the cell membrane, and when these are occupied by GABA chloride ions enter, the cell acquires a negative electrical potential and inhibition of the neuronal activity occurs.

In the early 1970s intense interest was stimulated by the discovery of certain endogenous brain substances, known collectively as ligands. The pain-relieving and anxiety-reducing effects of the opiates were known to be due to their ability to bond with receptor sites in the central nervous system but why such receptors for these drugs should exist remained a mystery until the discovery of the endogenous opioid ligands in the nervous system, the endorphins and enkephalins. The discovery of benzodiazepine (BZ) receptor sites was independently announced in the year 1977 by Squires and Braestrup and by Mohler and Okada; as yet no endogenous benzodiazepine-like substance has been identified. However, there are naturally occurring substances which bind with the BZ receptor sites but are antagonist in their action to benzodiazepine drugs and will reverse the hypnotic effect of a benzodiazepine overdose. The first to be discovered, by Braestrup and his colleagues, was extracted from human urine and is β-carboline-3-carboxylic acid ethyl ester or β-CCE. When a similar β-carboline derivative is administered to human volunteers it produces effects resembling the experience of anxiety.

Benzodiazepine receptors are widely distributed in the central nervous system and the highest density is in the phylogenetically younger areas of the brain such as the cerebral cortex, although subcortical areas such as the hippocampus and the amygdala also contain relatively high densities. There seem to be at least two distinct types of BZ receptor, with the BZ_1 receptor concentrated in the amygdaloid complex, the hippocampal formation and the prefrontal cortex. The BZ_1 receptors seem to determine anticonflict effects (at any rate in rats) and the BZ_2 receptors may be related to anxiety. Benzodiazepine drugs have a complex series of effects: they are sedatives (hypnotics in larger dose), they have anticonvulsant effects and in the animal laboratory they promote normal feeding activity in rats whose feeding responses were previously disrupted by electric shock (the 'anticonflict' effect). It is an article of clinical faith that they also have a true 'anxiolytic' effect and it is for this, and also because of their established dependence effects, that the phenomenon of widespread prescription exists. However, this anxiolytic effect is of short duration since tolerance rapidly develops and people continue to be anxious whilst consuming large quantities of the drugs; indeed, Braestrup and Nielson warned against the uncritical extrapolation from an anticonflict effect in rats to anxiolytic activity in man.

PHARMACOLOGICAL FACTORS

Study of the chemical neurotransmitters and the effects of drugs upon these, is leading to observations of relevance to an understanding of the phenomenon of anxiety. Several substances or procedures have been shown to induce the specific form of panic anxiety accompanied by sympathetic β-adrenergic overactivity in patients suffering from panic disorder. These substances include caffeine, the drug yohimbine, isoproterenol and inhalation of carbon dioxide. Caffeine is the most widely consumed psychotropic substance in the world and is well known for its stimulant effect; it is precisely in order to remain alert that people drink coffee and tea but only recently has it been observed that people who consume high doses of caffeine may develop symptoms of anxiety and that patients who suffer from panic disorder are sensitive to even small doses of caffeine. Yohimbine is an α_2-adrenergic antagonist interfering with noradrenergic transmission in the locus coeruleus and it provokes anxiety although the precise mechanism of action is not yet fully understood.

The effect of carbon dioxide (CO_2) on the nervous system is complex. A single inhalation of CO_2 may provoke a panic attack but lowering of the blood CO_2 level by hyperventilation provokes tetany with feelings of faintness and apprehension as well as the characteristic paraesthesiae and muscular spasm. The view now is that anxiety is enhanced by cognitive interpretation of feelings of bodily discomfort: thus the patient prone to panic attacks experiences a palpitation, fears that he may be about to have an attack or in some way lose control, and so anxiety spirals upwards to result in the full-blown panic attack. The same mechanism has been proposed for the anxiety-inducing effect of sodium lactate infusions.

The mechanism whereby imipramine and other tricyclic antidepressant drugs as well as the monoamine oxidase inhibiting drugs reduce and block panic attacks in panic disorder patients is not well established. It appears to be a different mechanism to the modification of 5-HT uptake at the synaptic cleft, which is thought to be the mechanism of effect of tricyclic antidepressants in depressive disorder, and indeed there seems to be no close relationship betwen panic disorder and major depressive disorder. Long-term treatment with antidepressant drugs reduces β-adrenergic receptor sensitivity whilst enhancing responses to serotonergic and α-adrenergic stimulation.

GABA is the major inhibitory neurotransmitter in the central nervous system. Benzodiazepine receptors are coupled with the GABA receptors, predominantly at the synaptic contacts; BZ receptors are widely distributed in the brain but particularly in the cerebral cortex and the hippocampus. Benzodiazepine drugs occupy their receptors and enhance the activity of GABA leading to inhibition of neuronal excitability; this is the mechanism of their sedative and anti-convulsant activity. The claim that the drugs have a specific 'anxiolytic' effect separate from the depressant effect on the brain is widely believed but difficult to sustain in the face of the clinical fact that many people continue to be very anxious despite taking high doses of the drugs over long periods of time. Other central nervous system depressants, the barbiturates and carbamates may also produce their effect *via* an interaction with the BZ–GABA complex and therefore ultimately through GABA-mediated chloride permeability.

PHYSICAL DISEASE AND ANXIETY

Anxiety is an understandable reaction to physical illness and the consequent distress, pain, handicap and threat to life. However, in certain diseases anxiety or anxiety-like symptoms may be a direct expression of the morbid process. A consideration of these is necessary in the differential diagnosis of anxiety states.

Hypoglycaemia

Lowering of the blood sugar produces effects on the central nervous system and symptoms secondary to the stimulation of secretion of noradrenaline. The former group of symptoms are basically those of cerebral depression, confusion and coma, although convulsions may occur. Noradrenaline release produces the classical effects of sympathetic overactivity: anxiety, sweating, tachycardia but also tremor and hunger. The noradrenaline oversecretion effects are more common in very rapid fall of blood sugar and this may result from overdose of insulin or sulphonylurea drugs. Insulin-secreting tumours, insulinomas, are an uncommon cause and may be confirmed by a high plasma insulin–plasma glucose ratio.

Hyperthyroidism

Overactivity of the thyroid gland, as in Grave's disease, results in the symptoms of hyperthyroidism. Excessive ingestion of thyroid hormone will produce the same effects. The symptoms are anxiety, insomnia, excessive sweating and intolerance of heat, frequent bowel movements, loss of weight despite a good appetite and weakness; women may have reduced or absent menstruation. The characteristic signs are a warm, moist skin, tremor, brisk reflexes and the characteristic eye signs of exophthalmos so that the white sclera is apparent above the pupil in normal forward vision, lid lag when following a downward moving object and failure to wrinkle the brow in upward gaze. Diagnosis is confirmed by thyroid function tests.

Phaeochromocytoma

Chromaffin tumours produce excess catecholamines and are most often located in the adrenal medulla itself. Paroxysmal hypertension is the essential feature and the attacks will probably be accompanied by other evidence of excessive sympathetic overactivity and the characteristic sense of anxiety which this induces. Diagnosis is confirmed by raised catecholamines in a 24-hour urine specimen.

Carcinoid Syndrome

Carcinoid tumours produce serotonin (5-HT) and other biologically active agents. There is characteristic flushing of the skin accompanied by tachycardia and these signs may be provoked by exertion, excitement, food or alcohol. Diagnosis is confirmed by the finding of increased urinary excretion of the serotonin metabolic product 5-hydroxyindole acetic acid (5-HIAA).

Cardiac Disorders

The sudden onset of tachycardia or runs of extrasystoles secondary to conduction disorders or disease of the myocardium will produce an uncomfortable sense of palpitation with secondary anxiety. It was recently stated that there was an association between mitral valve prolapse and panic disorder but further evaluation has confirmed that this is probably chance association of two commonly occurring conditions.

Ictal Disorders

Epileptic aura phenomena, especially in the temporal lobe, have a varied presentation of symptoms. Anxiety is the most prominent of the emotions but depression of suicidal intensity, aggression and also states of ecstasy may occur. Anxiety may be accompanied by the epigastic aura, which is a sensation of swelling arising from the abdomen towards the throat; this is the 'globus hystericus' and its occurrence gave rise to the ancient idea that the uterus took leave of its moorings in the pelvis. The notion is expressed in Shakespeare's King Lear:

> 'O how his mother swells up toward
> my heart! *Hysterica passio*
> Down thou climbing sorrow
> Thy element's below.'

The observation that strong emotion is associated with disturbance of the limbic area of the brain is thus long foreshadowed. The other phenomena associated with epileptic foci in this area of the brain are: depersonalization and derealization; distortions of time perception and experience of familiarity (*déjà vu*) or strangeness (*jamais vu*); distortions of the perception of the size of the body; hallucinations of oneself (autoscopic), Lilliputian hallucinations and hallucinations of taste and smell; forced thinking, i.e. the compulsive dwelling on a theme such as death or eternity.

During the fit the individual may be observed to make smacking movements with his mouth or twitch his nose in response to the hallucinated taste and smell. Diagnosis may be aided by special electroencephalographic techniques.

Withdrawal States

Withdrawal states from alcohol and drugs of dependency may be dominated by anxiety, especially when the withdrawal is rapid. Considering the extent of consumption of benzodiazepine drugs, drug withdrawal must be a major diagnostic consideration when states of anxiety occur 'inexplicably' in people admitted urgently to hospitals, prisons or other situations and their habitual medication has been abruptly stopped. Withdrawal states occur rapidly in people heavily dependent on alcohol and opiates. In the alcohol dependence syndrome effects occur whenever the blood alcohol level falls, as during sleep, and the person awakes with a feeling of fear, restlessness, tremulousness ('shakes'), nausea and sweating. More profound states and prolonged withdrawal will lead to vivid hallucinations, fits and delirium (delirium tremens). Opiate withdrawal is marked by vomiting and diarrhoea, abdominal cramps, muscle pains, sweating, running nose and eyes, dilated pupils, raised pulse and piloerection ('cold turkey' effect). Benzodiazepine withdrawal is less predictable, less violent in its manifestations and slower in onset. If the drugs are withdrawn suddenly from an individual who has been taking a large dose continuously for several

Table 3.1 Withdrawal manifestations

Benzodiazepines	Opiates	Alcohol
Anxiety insomnia	Anxiety insomnia	Anxiety insomnia
Muscle cramps	Muscle pains, cramps	Tremulousness
Nausea, retching	Vomiting, diarrhoea	Nausea, retching
Paraesthesia	Sweating	Sweating
Sensitivity to light, noise	Lachrymation	Hallucinations
Sense of motion	Piloerection	Epileptic fits
Hallucinations	Dilated pupils	
Epileptic fits	Epileptic fits	
Irritability		

months, rebound anxiety will usually occur together with any of the combination of symptoms listed in Table 3.1. Short-acting drugs such as lorazepam are particularly likely to produce withdrawal effects. In the case of the benzodiazepines these states may last for weeks, even months, after withdrawal. Relief following further prescription of the drug is a diagnostic test.

FURTHER READING

Gray, J. A. Anxiety as a paradigm case of emotion. *Brit Med Bull* 1981; **37**: 193–197.
Braestrup, C. and Nielson, M. Anxiety. *Lancet* 1982; **2**: 1030–1034.
Torgersen, Svenn. Genetic factors in anxiety disorders. *Arch Gen Psychiat* 1983; **40**: 1085–1089.
Tyrer, Peter. *The Role of Bodily Feelings In Anxiety*. Oxford: Oxford University Press, 1976.

Chapter 4

Psychological and Social Aspects of Anxiety: Causes and Effects

This chapter concerns itself with where anxiety comes from, the social situation in which it occurs, and where it is going to. We will consider aetiology in a broad sense, and prognosis.

Most of the interest in anxiety states and their related syndromes has been directed towards their physical and psychological aspects. Organic causes have been searched for and the individual psychological state thoroughly explored. Generally, social aspects have not commanded so much attention, perhaps because they have got themselves separated from the study of anxiety; the term stress has tended to be used more often in the social context. Anxiety and stress are, however, very closely connected. Theories of aetiology of the anxiety disorders may be physical, psychological or social. It is also necessary to consider the situations in which anxiety occurs, and also its course and prognosis. Physical aspects have been discussed in Chapter 3.

THEORIES OF AETIOLOGY

To understand the causes of anxiety disorders one needs not only to study the antecedents in the particular individual but also to know how it is that the experience of severe anxiety has come to be regarded as illness or disorder. This entails therefore both an understanding of the historical background and conceptualization of anxiety states (Chapter 2) and also knowledge of how they are classified and related to other physical and psychiatric disorders. Until one has set the nosological entity of anxiety states within the context of their classification, one cannot admit an individual patient to it. The aetiology of generalized anxiety is different from phobic states in that the latter are precipitated by specific objects or circumstances. However, phobic states may begin in the setting of more generalized anxiety or depression or both.

40

Early Upbringing and Child Rearing

In the first half of this century theories on the aetiology of neuroses including anxiety states were dominated by **psychoanalysis** as described by Freud and his followers. Psychoanalysis is a complex theory to describe abnormal functioning of the mind derived originally from the presentation of cases in clinical practice. Because psychoanalytic theory can be used to explain any behaviour both of the observed and the observer, it is not accessible to the fundamental requirements of scientific exploration, **falsification** and **verification**.

The information upon which psychoanalytic investigation is based is obtained from enquiry of the patient, particularly in the area of his current thoughts and fantasies, his dreams and the memories he can recall of his childhood experiences. **Free association** was found to be a useful method of helping the patient to reveal otherwise unconscious material. The patient is asked to say what first comes into his head in response to a stimulus word or idea. The analyst allows the 'client' to develop these associations gradually to reveal material that was not otherwise available to him. The analyst then suggests interpretations based upon psychoanalytic theory and the 'client' is invited to examine and accept or reject these interpretations.

As was discussed in Chapter 2, many of Freud's ideas had already been proposed centuries before he gathered them into a comprehensive explanatory theory.

Fundamental to Freud's explanations for neurotic illness was his concept that all mental processes originate at an **unconscious** level. Censorship takes place so that some of the mental content is made aware freely in consciousness, for example sensations. Some material only occasionally becomes conscious, for example memories which would be regarded as being in the preconscious mind. Some mental material is excluded altogether from consciousness — so the unconscious mind is separated from reality in that it contains gross contradictions, and it synthesizes the juxtaposition of events and experiences which actually occurred at very different times. Unconscious mind is dominated by the dynamic force of **libido**, which is the energy of the sexual instinct; this Freud regarded as being the underlying force for all subsequent activity. Freud believed there to be conflict between the powerful forces of the unconscious mind and the expression of the personality in consciousness.

It was postulated that repression into the unconscious allowed widely different unpleasant experiences to become associated and hence a phobia could arise from what appeared to be a relatively minor immediate provocation. Unconscious sexual urges were prevented from gaining expression throughout childhood by the implicit controls in the process of upbringing in society. The strength of the libido and the conflict between the drives of the unconscious mind and what was permitted to become manifest through the censorship of the superego resulted in the subjective experience of anxiety.

Freud postulated that anxiety could be reduced by various defence mechanisms. Using the technique of hypnosis and free association, Freud found that his patients showed resistance to remembering painful past events. This mechanism was called **repression** and the painful memories could be replaced by psychological or physical symptoms. The memory for the event and the emotion associated with it had become inaccessible to conscious thought through repression but it was still capable of influencing the roots of the person's thinking and behaviour at an unconscious level. Freud considered that sexual conflicts occurring in early childhood became frustrated in reaching consciousness and gaining expression, and this resulted in anxiety experienced in consciousness. In this theory, pathological anxiety is in fact failure of repression in that unacceptable impulses, desires and memories from an unconscious level are repressed; however, the libido may overcome the repression and present in consciousness in altered form resulting in anxiety symptoms or perhaps a panic attack. Later Freud developed the concept of **signal anxiety**, in which anxiety occurs and demonstrates to the self that the individual is in a position of danger. This then results in repression, which acts to reduce the level of anxiety and to achieve avoidance of the dangerous situation.

In Freud's *Studies in Hysteria* he describes the analysis of a case of panic state. Whilst walking in the Alps he met Katharina at the top of a mountain. She was aged 18 and, on ascertaining that Freud was a doctor, she told him about her symptoms: 'It suddenly comes upon me. There is first a pressure on my eyes. My head becomes so heavy and it hums so that I can hardly bear it, and then my chest begins to press together so that I cannot get my breath . . . the throat becomes laced together as if I choked . . . I always feel "now, I must die", and I am otherwise courageous, I go everywhere alone, into the cellar and down over the whole mountain, but on the day that I have this attack, I do not trust myself anywhere. I always believe that someone stands behind me and suddenly grabs me'. In psychological exploration, still taking place on the mountain, Freud discovered that the woman had been abused sexually by her uncle from about the age of 14. Katharina lived with her aunt, who because of a subsequent infidelity had recently divorced this uncle, and Katharina felt herself to be responsible for the marital breakdown. Freud regarded this repressed memory of **sexual trauma** as being the cause of her anxiety and current panic attacks.

Attachment Theory

Theories of attachment have arisen from a constructive synthesis of the work of the **object relations theorists** such as Fairbairn, Guntrip, Winnicott and Balint with the psychological and ethological studies of Harlow with the mothering of infant chimpanzees, Lorenz with emprinting and bonding, most dramatically amongst ducklings, Tinbergen with the development of chronic fear in autism, and Hinde with the effect of loss of mother on infant rhesus macaques in a stable social group. Bowlby has drawn these different strands together in his theory of maternal deprivation. He considers that if the maximal attachment with the mother between the child's age from nine months to three years is disrupted by separation, for instance due to mother leaving home or either mother or child going into hospital, then the child develops anxiety about the reliability of attachment figures. The later development of chronic anxiety could be seen as persistence of the emotions of separation and the threat of loss. Failure of attachment in the crucial intermediate phase of mother–child relationships may result in perpetual fear of the breakdown of relationships and loss of loved object, with generalized all-pervasive anxiety.

Learning Theory

This theory postulates that neurotic symptoms, like all other patterns of human behaviour, may be **learned** according to certain fixed principles. The mechanisms of learning were first described by Pavlov in the 1920s with the model of **classical conditioning**. In the simplest example of this, an unconditional stimulus will be followed by an appropriate response; for example, food placed in the mouth is followed by salivation. If a conditional stimulus is then repeatedly presented just before this unconditional stimulus, the response will eventually be produced by the conditional stimulus alone; for instance, regularly shining a light before presentation of food will after a number of combined applications produce salivation with the light alone. If the conditional stimulus is no longer paired with the unconditional stimulus, extinction of the conditional response eventually occurs: that is, salivation occurring after shining the light alone will in time cease to happen.

Pavlov's work on the causation of neurosis followed a flood in the animal house in Leningrad in which his experimental dogs were nearly drowned and became absolutely terrified. Water, even in small amounts, became for some of these animals a stimulus with the response of panic. Animal models have been used extensively for investigating the aetiology of neuroses but there is always, of course, doubt as to whether abnormality of behaviour in a laboratory animal is analogous to the experience of anxiety or other neurotic disorder in the human.

Classical conditioning may be used to explain an individual case. Where a conditional stimulus appears to have resulted in the response of anxious experience and behaviour, for example if sexual interest as a child is always punished, that person when adult may associate fear and anxiety with sexual arousal, with resultant anxiety and conflict in any sexually arousing situation. This simple model, however, does not fit the development of neuroses in humans in general. Explanations have been advanced as to the way in which the conditional stimulus has acquired **drive** properties, thus failing to result in extinction even though the unconditional stimulus is no longer presented.

Further animal work links the behavioural explanations for anxiety with phobia; for example, a laboratory animal may be taught to depress a lever to obtain food. After this behaviour has become established, depression of the lever is then accompanied by a conditional stimulus of an electric shock resulting in an unconditional response of pain. From this develops a conditional response of anxiety associated with pressing the lever. Avoidance of pressing may result; however, such a straightforward explanatory mechanism for the development of phobias in humans can only very rarely be demonstrated.

This type of explanation has also been used for the occurrence of panic disorder. A person may undergo a terrifying experience such as a threatened assault, and realization of his predicament results in tachycardia and tachypnoea, then a subjective feeling of intense anxiety and dread. The physiological symptoms may then become a conditional stimulus for the response of anxiety. Thus on a subsequent occasion when the individual has tachycardia, perhaps after physical exertion, acute anxiety and panic intervene. Again, the problem with this model is that panic disorder often occurs without such antecedents. It does not account for panic disorder continuing to occur despite the absence of further reinforcement. There is no clear evidence to support the theory that panic results from the perception of internal physiological change rather than a psychological evaluation of the situation itself.

The term **operant conditioning** was introduced by Skinner (1938) and assumes that behaviour is a voluntary response to a discriminative stimulus, that is, we determine what we will do and what choices we make according to the response we will get in terms of reward or punishment. Operant conditioning works on the principle of reinforcement. It is not difficult to see how the phobic behaviour of avoidance acts as a reinforcer in a situation where anxiety has become associated with certain circumstances. Avoidance of these circumstances results in relief of anxiety, thus strengthening the association of anxiety with the situation avoided.

Cognitive Aspects

Cognitive understanding of the causation of anxiety is based on the underlying theory that an individual's mood and behaviour are largely determined by the way in which s/he structures the world. His cognitions are the subjective events in his field of consciousness, either verbal or pictorial, and these are based upon attitudes or assumptions (otherwise called schemata) developed from previous experience. To illustrate this: two students are required to give a five-minute talk at a seminar. One student will approach this with considerable anxiety associated with an image of himself speaking hesitantly and drying up after two minutes; this is based upon very low self-esteem because of past failures. The other student, with self-confidence based on several rhetorical successes, may relish another opportunity for self-display.

In this theoretical approach to understanding different types of subjective emotion, the current affective state depends upon the person's own individual attitude to the world. With this aetiological theory the context within which the emotion of anxiety occurs is extremely important and one therefore needs to understand the individual's attitudes, why this situation creates fearful apprehension, and what are the earlier experiences that directed the person to this experience.

Anxiety is characterized by feelings of apprehension, uncertainty and helplessness associated with physiological changes. When anxiety is pathological these feelings occur without real external danger. Behaviour to avoid further anxiety is the usual response. Whereas with phobia there is a specific object or situation provoking anxiety, in generalized anxiety the apprehension is free-floating.

Personality and Personal Disorder

Discussing personality as an aetiological factor for the anxiety disorders begs the questions: what is personality in this context? and, what factors are aetiological for personality disorder?

Personality is the unique quality of the individual, his feelings and personal goals. It is seen in the characteristic pattern of behaviour of the individual; what makes him different from other people; the way we can predict he will act in any particular circumstances. It is manifested in social relationships including that between the patient and the clinician. When one or more traits of personality are present to an exceptional extent — more or less than usual — then personality is considered abnormal. If this abnormality of personality causes the person himself or other people to suffer, then personality disorder is said to be present.

The factors that mould personality and determine whether disorder occurs are broadly those that govern the presentation of neuroses: **constitutional** including both **genetic** and the **physical constitution; early upbringing, family and social environment and external circumstances** and **social disadvantage**. This is not the place to expatiate on such an enormous topic.

When assessing a person with anxiety disorder the personality should always be taken into account and this is an important clinical skill. The most appropriate classifications of personality disorder for medical use are typological in nature — that is, a constellation of traits or characteristics present in the individual to an abnormal extent, a personality **type**. There are several such lists of types in common use but that contained in Table 4.1, based upon the 9th Revision of the International Classification of Diseases, is useful because it is generally comprehensible.

Anxiety disorder is more frequent in those who show personality disorder. It is particularly likely to occur with affective personality disorder of anxious type, that is, **trait anxiety**; it is also common with anankastic, hysterical and asthenic personality disorders. Personality is an important factor in the manifestation of anxiety disorders which is often overlooked.

Table 4.1   Types of personality (based upon ICD 9)

301.0	Paranoid	Misconstrues others' personal rights, jealousy, self-importance, self-reference, fanatical, litiginous
301.1	Affective	Pronounced mood lifelong: depressive or elated, cyclothymic, anxious
301.2	Schizoid	Withdrawal, coolness and detachment
301.3	Explosive	Liability to intemperate outbursts of mood
301.4	Anankastic	Insecurity, doubt, conscientiousness, perfectionism, rigidity
301.5	Hysterical	Shallow, labile affect, appreciation craving, theatricality, sexual immaturity
301.6	Asthenic	Passive compliance, inadequacy, lack of vigour
301.7	Asocial	Lack of feeling for others, callous, cold, rejects social norms, irresponsible, does not learn from experience

SOCIAL DETERMINANTS

One of the earliest epidemiological studies of the neuroses was carried out by Taylor and Chave (1964) to investigate the health of a new town largely comprised of young families rehoused from London. Four symptoms of minor psychiatric disorder tended to cluster: 'nerves' (close to a generic concept of anxiety), depression, undue irritability and sleeplessness, and this constellation was called **subclinical neurosis syndrome**. Rates for these symptoms were broadly similar in the new town, an outer London housing estate and the inner London borough from which most of those who were rehoused originally came. Those with these symptoms were more likely than others to consider their health to be poor, more likely to be treated by their general practitioners for neurotic disorder, and more likely to consult their general practitioner with all types of complaint both physical and psychological.

Although these subjects had not lost contact with friends and relatives, they frequently complained of being lonely; they spent considerable time at home and disliked doing this; they had difficulty in making friends and this was due to lack of capacity rather than opportunity. Those who were neurotic were less likely to be satisfied with their environment.

Stress, as associated with anxiety, has been discussed in Chapter 1. Anxiety is the subjective description of an emotion that might be called, objectively, a **stress reaction**. Stress may be considered to occur when there is a lack of fit between the person and his environment. It is individual, and what is stressful for one person will not necessarily be so for another.

Work

Anxiety is commonly associated with problems in different life situations, such as stress at work. The threat of redundancy and subsequent unemployment has been shown to be associated with an increased consultation rate with the general practitioner for anxiety and related symptoms. This reaction, with symptoms resulting, occurs before the job is actually lost and sometimes with only a slight threat of future unemployment.

Occupational causes of anxiety have certainly been well recognized for more than 150 years (see Chapter 2). There is very considerable interest in this subject at the present time, with such expressions as 'executive stress' and 'burnout' being used in management parlance. Stress at work is associated to a greater extent with the expectations the individual has for himself and the way he interprets the demands of others upon him than with the physical environment of the place of work. Working relationships are also very important in creating situations of stress, and in alleviating them. Relationship difficulties with consequent anxiety may occur with the worker's peers, with his superiors at work and with subordinates, and different factors may be operative in each of these situations.

Problems at work are likely to be perceived as more stressful by those with an existing anxiety state or other neurotic disorder. Such people will be less tolerant of bad working conditions such as noise, extremes of temperature, humidity, vibration or poor illumination, and neurotic symptoms such as phobia or anxiety may become linked to problems at work. Both fatigue and, contrarily, too little work are potent stresses. Work that is excessively boring may be perceived by the worker as stressful and result in anxiety; various devices have been introduced in industry more or less successfully to overcome the problem of the boredom of some work.

Losing one's employment, changing to a different type of work and retirement have all been found to be major **life events**. Loss of work is likely to increase the risk of both physical and psychiatric morbidity. Three phases in response to unemployment were identified 50 years ago. The first phase is shock, denial and also a sense of optimism — the individual may take what he regards as a long-deserved holiday; the second phase is distress, and this increases as the person finds it difficult to obtain work and experiences economic hardship; in the third phase he develops the 'unemployed identity', stops looking systematically for work and becomes haphazard and dispirited, hopeless about ever obtaining further employment. This latter manifests in this area of life the symptomatology of neurotic depression. Sometimes **threat** of loss of employment tends to provoke anxiety state, and actual **loss** of work, especially with long-term unemployment, to result in neurotic depression.

Marriage and Sex

Marital disharmony and sexual dysfunction may both result from and cause anxiety. Neurosis of all types is associated with marital discord, separation and divorce. Those who are neurotically predisposed have more difficulty in establishing a mutually satisfying marital relationship, and a discordant marriage is a potent precipitant of further neurotic reaction. Poor marital adjustment can be seen as an imbalance between caregiving and the need for attachment. It has been shown that where mental illness occurs within a marriage, most frequently a diagnosis of neurosis or personality disorder is made for the wife and alcoholism for the husband.

Anxiety is commonly associated with sexual pathology in the male or female. Anxiety concerning capacity for performance inhibits sexual behaviour, and past difficulties in sexual expression are major causes of anxiety. Anxiety and sexual dysfunction, then, becomes so closely intertwined that there can be no effective treatment for the dysfunction until anxiety has been dealt with adequately. Sexual tension is a potent cause of dysfunction with resultant deleterious effects upon the marriage.

Agoraphobia and social phobias are most common in young married women. This may to some extent be associated with the change of social environment that occurs when a young woman loses the social supports of her family of origin and moves to an area where she does not know her neighbours. She may now live in a district in the outer suburbs of the city whilst her mother remains in the inner city. Leaving her job and looking after young children necessarily restricts her capacity to go out of the house. She may perceive there to be an element of economic and social competitiveness with her neighbours, thus increasing her feeling of self-consciousness and also isolation.

Anxiety states are frequent under such circumstances. A common situation in psychiatric referral is for such a woman to present initially with agoraphobia, but as these symptoms remit in response to treatment and the patient becomes more confident in talking about herself, so marital problems which were originally denied become more prominent. Not infrequently the husband in such a marriage feels frustrated and isolated with his phobic, anxious, distressed wife but at the same time feels guilty in his inadequacy to do anything to improve her emotional state. This results in an escalating spiral of marital discord and a search for alternative sources of consolation such as alcohol or another partner.

Although the patient with marital problems may complain of symptoms of anxiety, other presentations are also frequent such as **psychosomatic symptoms** (physical symptoms without organic cause), sleep disorder, depression, or drug or alcohol abuse. Deliberate self-harm with overdosage of prescribed medication is common, and marital difficulty is very often given as the cause for self-poisoning. Anxiety problems associated with the marriage may also have roots in other social situations; thus the wife whose husband is promoted at work may experience anxiety when she is expected to make public appearances as his spouse. Alternatively, when both partners are working there may be competitiveness between them with consequent anxiety for the one who is less successful at work.

Anxiety may result from relationships with other family members such as parents-in-law. Problems in the marriage of parents is a precipitant for anxiety symptoms in the children. The anxiety, and especially specific phobias, of children may closely mirror those of one or other parent.

Psychological Trauma

The conditions under which people live, both short term and long term, have a lot to do with their development of anxiety states. Thus times of economic change and high unemployment have been discussed as provocations; so also are war and other major disasters. These conditions do not necessarily increase the frequency of neurotic breakdown in a defined population, but the content of the neurotic conflict, the way anxiety presents, reflects these background conditions.

Communicated Anxiety

Epidemic, communicated or mass neurosis may be transmitted to a large number of people, especially in a closed community. In this situation neurosis may be contagious in a psychological sense: that is, close contact with an individual who already has symptoms may result in the transmission of those symptoms to somebody previously unaffected. Anxiety symptoms are particularly likely to be conveyed in this way, and such symptoms include hyperventilation, fainting, parasthaesiae and other physical manifestations.

Such epidemics have been described throughout history. Spread occurs first *via* those who are most emotionally unstable and are already experiencing considerable conflict. Symptoms of overbreathing, dizziness, fainting, headache, shivering, pins and needles, nausea, pain in the back or abdomen, hot feelings and general weakness were described in an epidemic that spread through a school in Blackburn. In each class the epidemic first spread to young females of high status in the peer group who had particular problems at that time. As was discussed in Chapter 2, panic was originally considered to be a social and communicated emotion. The spread of terror through a group of individuals has been clearly described for other animal species as well as for humans.

MANIFESTATION OF ANXIETY

Not only do anxiety and anxiety disorders have an effect upon the individual, causing him to experience symptoms and discomfort (described as psychopathology in Chapter 5), but they also have an effect upon the subject's behaviour and hence upon the community and the society in which he lives. These social manifestations are often overlooked in medical and clinical psychological practice because the main emphasis is understandably and correctly based on the individual himself. However, the social manifestations of anxiety as they impinge upon the family and the wider community have repercussions for the individual because other people respond to him in a manner dictated by these social manifestations.

Talcott Parsons has pointed out that the effects physical illness has upon a person will be determined by sociological forces; society bestows a **sick role** upon people who are considered by that society to be ill. The components of this sick role are: (1) exemption from normal responsibilities of life; (2) exemption from responsibility for certain aspects of behaviour; (3) a responsibility to try to recover from the illness; and (4) a responsibility to seek appropriate health care. The term **illness behaviour** has been used by Mechanic to describe the activities that people undertake when they consider themselves to be ill. These include consultation with doctors, receiving medication, being treated by relatives and friends as sick, and refraining from certain activities such as work. If a state of anxiety is considered by the individual sufferer and by those around him to amount to a disorder, then his relatives may invest him with a sick role and he may take on illness behaviour; this may be appropriate in getting rid of his symptoms or alternatively may in fact prolong the state of disability. There are disadvantages in labelling a subjective state or item of behaviour as illness or disease in that it may result in the individual himself or his peers maintaining him in that state.

Somatic symptoms are a prominent feature of anxiety states and usually demonstrate abnormality of autonomic activity such as palpitations or diarrhoea or increased muscle tension such as headache, chest pain or backache. Hyperventilation will result in secondary symptoms of hypocapnia such as dizziness, paraesthesiae and feeling faint. This combination of palpitations, pain in the chest (usually in the chest wall) and hyperventilation and its consequences was in the past described as effort syndrome or **disorderly action of the heart**. This became associated with other cardiac illness, and hence patients with these symptoms were referred to the cardiological clinic. Such patients sometimes presented with chronic morbidity, and there was gross restriction of activity due to failure to make a diagnosis. Sometimes chronic physical symptoms of this kind demonstrate how chronic anxiety is both reinforced by and nurtures the physical symptoms that occur.

It needs to be borne in mind that humans do not only convey meaning with words and language; they also communicate non-verbally. This is also true with the physical manifestations of anxiety, for example tremor or hyperventilation may eloquently express the patient's distress or fear and may serve this purpose unconsciously or deliberately to reveal the individual's inner feelings to a doctor or other health professional. Anxiety symptoms may therefore act as a form of signalling.

Stress and adverse life experiences may be seen not only as aetiological explanations for the occurrence of anxiety but also as ways in which anxiety manifests. The person who is currently anxious because of trait anxiety arising from an underlying affective personality or acute anxiety reaction is much more vulnerable to the disorders normally associated with stress. This may show itself in the realm of work and unemployment, in marriage and the family or in the individual's social network. In studying the relationship between the individual and society it is important not only to assess the effects of society upon the individual but also how the characteristics of the individual modify those effects.

The **social network** has been studied by Scott Henderson and co-workers, proposing the hypothesis that a deficiency in social relationships is a causal factor in the onset of neuroses or non-psychotic disorders. **Anophelia** was defined as a state of real or perceived deficiency in relationships and this was considered to be aetiological in neurosis irrespective of whether there were also adverse circumstances or not.

The social network is a way of conceptualizing social relationships and depends upon Bowlby's concept of attachment for a theoretical basis. When considering the persons and the provisions of the network, it was seen that relationships had to be both available and adequate, and assessment of these independently became the basis of measurement in the Interview Schedule for Social Interaction. Attachments and social integration were measured separately, assessing each for both availability and adequacy of relationships. People suffering from anxiety or depression show prominent disturbance in social relationships as measured on this scale. Figure 4.1 shows comparison at long-term follow-up of a population previously treated for severe neurotic disorder with a normal population (comprised of people treated for varicose veins in the same year) on a measure of outcome which is mainly social in its construction. The neurotic group shows great disadvantage in this area.

Anxiety and Culture

It has been described above how anxiety may be communicated by contagion. That is, the cause of anxiety in person B may be the closeness of the contact with person A who experienced acute anxiety prior to B. The particular characteristics of the person's own culture and individual society are highly relevant.

It is important for an individual human being to have a sense of belonging to a group or society: '**integration** into a group, and the integrity of the self, are linked concepts. In one ancient language, the noun for "home" is the same word as the verb "I am"' (Rack). Loss of this sense of belonging results in

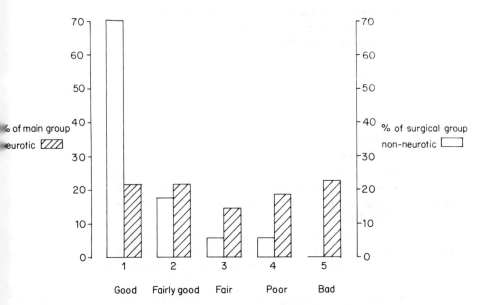

Figure 4.1: Total outcome at follow-up — neurotic group compared with surgical group

dislocation, a sense of loss and all-pervasive anxiety. This may be associated with migration and is especially likely for refugees who leave their home out of extreme fear. Consequent anxiety may take the form of irrational behaviour and feelings of extreme fear, hate, or alternatively irrational affection; such people may become intensely dependent upon those around them, sometimes quite casual acquaintances. Others will respond to their anxiety with dissociative experiences and a retreat into fantasy. The experience of migration has much in common with other experiences of loss such as bereavement, and it may go through similar stages of numbness, separation anxiety and despair. Homesickness is described not infrequently by elderly immigrants even 50 years after leaving their original home. Such adverse emotions of anxiety or misery may be rekindled after many years of good adjustment by, for example, bad news from their home country.

Both depression and anxiety may be obscured by physical symptoms taking precedence over the psychological state—**somatization**. This may be partly linguistic in nature but also reflects, quite realistically, what the patient expects from the doctor and expects the doctor to take an interest in. Patients know from experience that doctors are likely to take more notice of an unpleasant symptom in the chest than a description of feeling frightened. It has been suggested that in some languages there is a lack of words to describe dysphoria. However, on more careful analysis these words are usually found to be present but not to be in the currency offered to the doctor. In western Europe, by contrast, it is important to realize that somatic symptoms are an essential component of the expression of anxiety.

Distinct cultural descriptions of anxiety occur in which particular symptoms cluster in a characteristic manner; for example, **latah** is a form of communicated neurosis which has a number of different names and slightly different forms in various communities in South East Asia. Characteristic is hypersuggestibility, automatic obedience, speaking obscenities out loud, and various echo phenomena. It has been described as occurring particularly in lower social class women exposed to sudden overwhelming stress associated with war, natural disasters or drastic social change. It is therefore a form of post-traumatic or aftermath neurosis.

In **koro**, occurring in Chinese communities, there is extreme fear that the penis will shrink back into the abdomen and cause the patient to die. It is associated with considerable terror and the sufferer may hold onto his penis to prevent what he believes to be the inevitable consequences. **Susto** occurs in South America and describes temporary loss of the soul from the body as a result of acute stress. **Jiryan** is a fixed belief that sperm is leaking from the body in the urine. This symptom of anxiety occurs in Pakistan and is associated with the belief that sperm is formed from blood and that neither blood nor sperm are renewable: therefore once lost, there is a permanent diminution in potency causing anxiety, fear and guilt.

Extreme symptoms of anxiety have often been associated with the belief by the sufferer that he or she is bewitched. This is very commonly associated with

voodoo; in Haiti the symptoms are often described in equestrian terms in which the spirit is regarded as the rider and the suffering human as the horse.

The **brain fag** syndrome has been described predominantly in Africa and is a culturally specific form of persistent anxiety. It occurs particularly in the member of an uneducated family sent, because of signs of early promise, for further education. Academic failure may result in anxiety, shame at the anticipated confrontation by the family and hence further anxiety resulting in rapidly deteriorating academic performance. The sufferer will describe a variety of physical symptoms including headache and difficulty with vision; of course, problems with concentration and with study are prominent,

Aftermath Neurosis (Post-Traumatic Stress Disorder)

Post-traumatic stress disorder or **aftermath neurosis** commonly presents with anxiety symptoms. Being a victim in a catastrophe is extremely stressful and has a massive short-term and long-term effect upon mental equilibrium. Two mechanisms explaining the emotional reactions in major disaster are: first, the experience of loss with loss of health, loss of property, loss of relatives, loss of status, and so on, is known to provoke neurotic reaction; second, the experience of being involved in the collective drama of the catastrophe also appears to be associated with an increased degree of neurotic reaction.

The greater the degree of involvement with the disaster, the more likely is there to be anxiety and other symptoms and also a feeling of separation from the larger community who are not involved. Following such involvement in major disaster, even without actual physical injury, long-term neurotic disability may occur with phobic anxiety symptoms, irritability and depression protracted over many months, and sometimes for years. Such symptoms were described in the uninjured victims of a bomb-blast. There was also an increase in some subjects from moderate levels of alcohol intake to established dependence. These victims often described deterioration in marital relationships and with employment, both ascribed to their reaction to the experience of bombing.

Distinct stages in the reaction to disaster have been described (Figure 4.2). These are: preimpact, warning, impact, recoil and postimpact or aftermath. Various degrees and expressions of anxiety may occur at each of these stages. During the **Preimpact** stage, in a state of heightened awareness of the possibility of danger in a community, certain individuals may have a degree of anxiety that paralyses effective action. At the **warning** stage, a few hours before the disaster, when in some instances it is possible to take avoiding action, a certain level of anxiety is beneficial, but excessive anxiety will prevent any effective action. If the **impact** is protracted, anxiety is a normal and universal reaction.

In the **recoil** stage different types of emotional reaction may be shown by the victims. They may be numbed and apathetic, they may show acute panic reactions, or they may show inappropriate apathetic and automatic behaviour. In the **postimpact** or aftermath stage certain individuals, especially those who were for reasons of previous neurotic illness or social difficulty more vulnerable, may

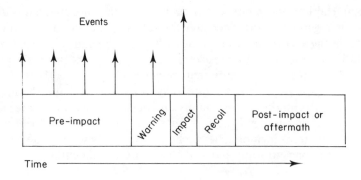

Figure 4.2: Stages of psychological reaction to disaster

show prolonged neurotic reaction; this may be a chronic anxiety state and a persistent reexperiencing of the traumatic events either in daytime fantasy or in nightmares.

Alcohol and Drug Misuse

There is a complex relationship between anxiety and **substance misuse**. Alcohol, for example, is a powerful anxiolytic agent, and a common form of misuse begins with the discovery that alcohol in small dosage at times of stress will reduce discomfort and perhaps improve social performance, or at any rate relieve the distress the subject experiences in acknowledging his performance to be impaired by anxiety. In the past barbiturates, and currently benzodiazepine drugs, have been used by patients and prescribed by doctors for the same purpose. The problem with the use of alcohol for this purpose is that it becomes habit-forming and also that tolerance develops in that a larger amount of the drug is required to achieve the same effect. This may eventually result in dependence.

Withdrawal of habit-forming anxiolytic drugs such as alcohol or benzodiazepines may result in increasing and persistent anxiety. This may be due to a return of the anxiety to reduce which the drug was taken in the first place or it may be a direct withdrawal symptom; in practice, where such a drug has been taken in moderate dosage for some time, probably both these factors are in operation. This unpleasant result of reduction in dose is the reason, from the individual's point of view, to maintain the drug in the present amount.

Anxiety may also be experienced while the individual remains on a constant dose of alcohol or anxiolytic drug. This may be associated with the social consequences of alcohol abuse, such as family or work problems. Alternatively, anxiety may be experienced, especially in those with neurotic predisposition, when taking small doses of benzodiazepine drugs the individual believes himself to have become addicted to. This anxiety, when associated with the genuine pharmacological effects of the drug, increases the difficulty in reducing the dosage of medication.

Anxiety is occasionally described as a reason for self-poisoning or other form of deliberate self-harm such as wrist-slashing. The individual describes experiencing an unbearable state of tension which is temporarily relieved by this activity.

Mind Persuasion

Mental coercion or brainwashing has been used throughout history to achieve conformity and also to extract confessions. Such methods have been developed systematically, using psychological insights, over the last half century following Van Der Lubbe's forced confession to burning down the Reichstag building in 1933 and then later during the Moscow purge trials in the late 1930s and during the Korean War.

An elaborate system of indoctrination is used to achieve 'conversion' and self-accusation resulting in total submission and acquiescence by concentration upon the feelings of guilt that are already latent inside the individual and by creating a sense of uncertainty with loss of any expectation of relief and removal of all hope for the future. The victim is kept isolated and drugs, sensory deprivation and torture have been used to increase the feelings of terror and pain. The victim is trained to accept and believe his confession and that of others, and this is rehearsed continuously. He is also persuaded to make full statements about other people. This form of neurosis provoked by extreme stress is associated with overwhelming feelings of anxiety, fear and despair. Such individuals are likely to experience long-term and probably permanent sequelae of depression and anxiety after release from their ordeal.

OUTCOME OF ANXIETY DISORDERS

Having discussed the different theories that may account for the occurrence of various types of anxiety and the social situations which may be associated with its manifestations, we will now look at the natural history of these conditions.

Factors predictive of outcome in neurotic disorders are shown in Figure 4.3; most of these are applicable to anxiety and phobic neuroses. Duration of symptoms at the time of interview is certainly predictive in that long-established disability is likely to be followed by chronic anxiety state. The outcome for the severe and established cases of anxiety and phobic neurosis seen in psychiatric practice is not benign. Persisting neurotic symptoms and quite marked social impairment were frequent when those suffering initially from relatively severe neurotic disorder were compared at 12-year follow-up with a sample of people who did not suffer from neurotic symptoms. At follow-up 90 per cent of the non-neurotic group were found to have a satisfactory outcome as far as symptoms, requirement for treatment over the intervening years, the development of alcohol and drug dependence and any evidence of social disruption were concerned; however, only 44 per cent of the previous neurotic group had done as well.

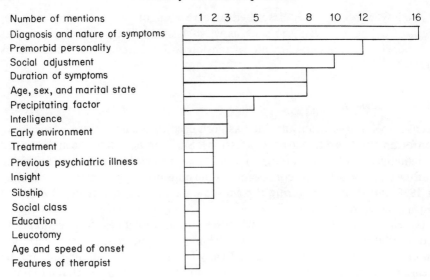

Figure 4.3: Factors mentioned as predictive of outcome in follow-up studies of neuroses

Dependence upon drugs, alcohol, tobacco and also upon other people is commonly found when these more severe sufferers from anxiety and phobic states are followed up. In one study those who were suffering from a neurotic disorder without alcohol or drug dependence were followed up 12 years later. Ten per cent of these patients demonstrated established dependence on either alcohol or drugs as shown by the presence of withdrawal symptoms, problems arising from excessive consumption of drugs or alcohol, or deliberate self-harm using drugs. Those who have become dependent upon drugs or alcohol have a worse outcome than others. There is also an association between dependence among these patients and abnormality of personality.

There is an association between smoking and anxiety in that those who are smokers are more likely to light up when they are feeling anxious or stressed. A survey of the smoking habits of patients suffering from neurotic disorders was carried out and compared with a surgical control group from the same hospital and also with general population surveys. Neurotic patients were more likely to be smokers than others; those neurotic subjects who smoked consumed more cigarettes per day than non-neurotic smokers; they tended to start smoking at a younger age; and they were more likely to inhale deeply.

Over the years, those suffering from chronic anxiety and phobic neuroses are more likely to become emotionally dependent upon other people including their general practitioners. They make frequent attendance at surgery with multiple complaints, and a variety of symptomatic treatments have often been prescribed. There is also frequent referral to different hospital specialists. There is a substantial increase in uptake of general practitioner time by those suffering from anxiety disorders.

A somewhat unexpected finding, considering that there is no demonstrable organic disorder present, is that mortality is increased with anxiety disorders. Coryell and co-workers found an unexpectedly high death rate both from suicide and cardiovascular disease amongst a group of previously hospitalized patients suffering from panic disorder. It has been shown at follow-up that sufferers from neurotic disorders have a significantly increased mortality. The relative risk of death for all causes of death for these subjects was found to be 1.7, for suicide 6.8, for accidents 4.6, and for diseases of the nervous, respiratory and circulatory systems 1.6. The relative risk is the observed number of deaths divided by the expected number. As well as suicide and accidents there was a significantly increased mortality for natural causes. Amongst natural causes the most significant increase in deaths was from arteriosclerotic conditions such as hypertension, peripheral vascular disease and coronary artery disease. This may be associated with the observed increase in smoking by neurotic patients under stress as discussed above. There is very little known about the dietary habits or body configuration of anxious patients.

We do not have much information about the changes in frequency of anxiety, panic and phobic disorders over time or in different cultures. However, what information we do have tends to point more to the similarity of the frequency of different conditions, at different times and in different places rather than marked variation in frequency. The presentation of anxiety differs in other cultures, but it is probable that frequency does not vary substantially. Personality factors are, of course, important in the aetiology.

FURTHER READING

Henderson, S. *Neurosis in the Social Environment*. Sydney: Academic Press, 1981.
Rack, P. *Race, Culture and Mental Disorder*. London: Longmans, 1982.
Sims, A. C. P. *Neurosis in Society*. Basingstoke: MacMillan, 1983.
Taylor, S. J. and Chave, S. *Mental Health and Environment*. London: Longmans, 1964.

Chapter 5

The Psychopathology of Anxiety

THE SYMPTOMS OF ANXIETY STATES

The state of anxiety is manifest by symptoms in the domains of mood, thought or attitudes (cognitions) and somatic (bodily) disturbance. Disturbance in all three areas is not invariably present: for instance, a person may have somatic disturbance but deny experiencing anxious thoughts. Moreover there is a tendency to individual response style and one person may always develop tension pains in one area of the musculature, another may sweat when he becomes anxious and another person may not experience somatic symptoms although anxious cognitions are marked.

Anxious Mood

Anxiety has been called 'fear, spread out thin' and the characteristic of the anxious mood is a pervasive feeling of a fear which cannot be attributed to a cause, of apprehension of some nameless disaster. Anxious mood of morbid severity, especially when it occurs in acute bursts as in panic disorder (see below), is a state which can only be described by the word terror. Alongside the disorder of mood is the state of overarousal or abnormal vigilance; the person over-responds to slight noises or shadows, a state for which he may use the phrase 'jump out of my skin', and sleep is denied.

The Somatic Symptoms of Anxiety

These fall into two major groups: muscular tension, and a gamut of symptoms partly determined by variable activity of the limbic areas of the brain and the autonomic nervous system, especially its sympathetic division.

Taking muscular symptoms, different groups of the muscles may be affected and result in pains in any area of the body but characteristically the scalp muscles are affected and the result is 'tension headache'. The muscle tension pain tends to have a constant, nagging quality. Muscle tension is also experienced as a difficulty in relaxing, resulting in restlessness; the enormous expenditure of purposeless physical energy may lead to a sense of great fatigue. Tremor ma, occur, particularly in the hands, when the person is under observation and attempting an activity requiring fine coordination such as passing a full cup of tea to another person. Individual tics, spasms and cramps may occur but have many other causes.

The symptoms dependent upon limbic lobe activity may also occur in somatic disorder of the temporal lobe of the brain: a sense of unreality (depersonalization or derealization) and a sense of warmth rising upwards from the pelvic area through the body (globus hystericus). More common are the symptoms of autonomic nervous system overstimulation: palpitations, sweating, dry mouth, loss of appetite, overactivity of bowels, frequency and the sense of suffocation from which the word 'anxiety' is derived. The latter may lead to overbreathing and this may bring in train the symptoms of lowered arterial carbon dioxide resulting in tetany: paraesthesia (tingling), muscle cramps, faintness and, rarely, convulsions.

Cognitions

In a state of anxiety the person feels insecure and inadequate. He worries excessively and small problems assume the proportions of gigantic tasks. Thoughts revolve around the themes of safety in a manner which the person knows to be unrealistic but nonetheless his activities become hedged about by fear. Just as fear may be pervasive ('free-floating') or focused on a limited range of situations — phobias — so may worrying thoughts be pervasive or a single theme may predominate over all others.

THE CLASSIFICATION OF ANXIETY STATES

There is a tendency to divide up anxiety states into somewhat artificial groups in accord with prevailing ideas about causation and response to treatment. Tyrer (1984) has considered the merits and demerits of this procedure, which now reaches its apogee in the Revised version of the American *Diagnostic and Statistical Manual*, Vol. 3 (DSM IIIR). The DSM classification of anxiety disorders is:

- Generalized anxiety disorder
- Panic disorder, with agoraphobia
- Panic disorder, without agoraphobia
- Agoraphobia, without history of panic disorder
- Simple phobia
- Social phobia
- Obsessive compulsive disorder
- Post-traumatic stress disorder
- Anxiety disorder, not otherwise specified

There are some advantages in this system and the seemingly complicated sub-divisions of panic disorder and agoraphobia will be considered below. However, the defects include an absence of the concept of trait anxiety in abnormal degree: an anxious personality disorder. We will include this consideration. If social anxiety is to be considered as a separate entity there seems no reason to exclude other major domains of anxiety, especially illness fears and sexual anxiety. The inclusion of obsessive–compulsive disorder among the anxiety states is debatable. Obsessional symptoms may occur in the setting of generalized anxiety but more often have their origin in the setting of depressive states; we will not consider them here except to distinguish obsessional symptoms from phobias.

Trait Anxiety

There is probably a constitutional proneness to anxiety based upon genetic endowment. However, anxious people grow up in anxious families, therefore just how much anxiety is genetically based and how much is imbibed from the milieu of familial interrelationships and patterns of thought and behaviour becomes impossible to distinguish in any individual. Certainly being anxious becomes an extraordinarily enduring trait once established and many people will describe themselves as 'born worriers'. In such people, even with the most careful life history given by an observer who has known the person from an early age, it may be impossible to discern a time when he was not anxious, although stress may have interacted with a personal predisposition to produce a more acute anxiety state. This matter is emphasized since the proneness to the enduring trait of anxiety is an important consideration when planning an anxiety management therapeutic programme. (See Figure 5.1.)

> At the age of 32 Sarah was referred for advice about tension headache which was causing increasing absenteeism from work. She described a vague sense of apprehension at the beginning of every day and she worried about making some error in her clerical work and thereby losing business for the firm. All her life she had been shy, had never made close friends or married; she said she had not married because of her fear of having young children under her care. Her own childhood was made miserable by the noisy arguments between her parents and she recalled that, as a very young child, she would strive to remain awake until she knew her mother had gone safely to bed.

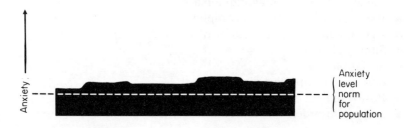

Figure 5.1: Trait anxiety

Generalized Anxiety Disorder

The commonest form of anxiety state commences in a gradual way in the setting of stress, conflict or uncertainty for the future well-being and security of the individual and his family or group. There is usually a background of proneness to anxiety (trait anxiety) or some other vulnerability of personality such as dependency and indecisiveness. However, an anxiety state may occur in a person with a robust personality structure if stress is prolonged and severe. The manifestations of the disorder are the mood of anxiety, anxious cognitions and somatic symptoms in variable degree. The extent to which anxiety is focused on certain situations with avoidance responses (phobias) is variable but typically the feeling of general insecurity leads to a wide range of low-grade avoidance of situations where such feelings are likely to be increased, such as crowds or being exposed to the possibility of criticism by others. The origin of the anxiety state is clear to the patient or, if it is not, he is usually able to accept an explanation of his state in terms of the interaction of stress and personality structure. Where this causal explanation is not so clear and when the severity of anxiety seems totally out of proportion to any stress, then an underlying biogenic depressive disorder should be suspected (see below). Anxiety states have a marked tendency to persist once the causative stress has been relieved or overcome and these are the cases for which effective anxiety management therapy is important if prolonged disability is not to be the sequel. (See Figure 5.2.)

A teacher was in a quandary as to whether to accept promotion in a substandard inner city school or to move to a new town where it would be hard to meet the expenses and his wife would have no employment to supplement the family income. He was aware of becoming tense but anxiety reached a morbid degree following the death of a pupil in a car accident. He was unable to sleep and when he did sleep his wife was kept awake by his tooth grinding. He irritated his son by overconcern for his safety, insisting that he must not leave the house after the evening meal. He had worried about illness as a child, for his father was admitted repeatedly to hospital with coronary thromboses. He had attempted to overcome these fears by forcing himself to read stories about hospitals and imagining himself as a doctor or ambulance driver dealing with fearful emergencies; but in these fantasies he always made mistakes and the patient died.

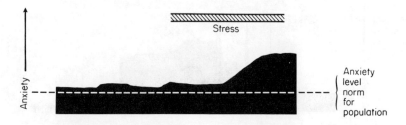

Figure 5.2: Stress-induced state anxiety

Panic Disorder

In contrast to the generalized anxiety disorder this state commences abruptly, and frequently precipitating stress is absent or of low degree and of the type which the person has previously experienced without developing anxiety of such alarming intensity. There may have been no major flaws in the personality structure and no preceding psychiatric illness. It typically commences in young adults, and women are more prone to the disorder than men. There is a sudden unheralded mood of intense fear accompanied by any of a wide range of somatic symptoms of anxiety but most commonly severe palpitation, choking sensation, paraesthesia (tingling sensations), dizziness, faintness, flushing and sweating. The experience is so alarming and so inexplicable that the person may think he is about to die or become insane; he is likely to summon a doctor or have himself rushed to a hospital emergency department where physical examination reveals no abnormality. After an hour or two the attack subsides but after an interval of a few days or a few weeks another attack occurs, and then another, and the effect of these further attacks is to leave the patient with a raised level of generalized anxiety. (See Figure 5.3.)

Another common sequel is the development of avoidance responses; these may be limited to just a few specific situations or there may be a wide range. The patient fears approaching the situation in which he experienced his first panic attack; for instance, if this occurred in a department store he is understandably apprehensive about entering the store, or similar building, again. Then, if the next attack occurred whilst travelling on a bus he becomes frightened of bus transport and if the next attack occurs when walking in the park he is consequently frightened of wide-open spaces. Now the underlying panic disorder with the spontaneous unprovoked attacks may subside, as it generally does after a few months, but a range of avoidance responses of situations remains as a long-term aftermath. Any attempt to enter the feared situation causes severe apprehension as the patient recollects the former agonizing panic attack. This is the so-called 'agoraphobic' syndrome (misnamed because it is not just a fear of market places); in the worst outcome the patient may be virtually housebound, and even in the 'safety' of his own home he may be terrified at the prospect

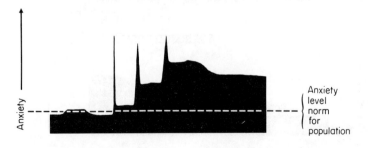

Figure 5.3: Panic disorder

of being left on his own. The level of generalized anxiety is very much higher in patients suffering from agoraphobia than in patients who have simple phobias of single situations such as moths, hypodermic needles or thunderstorms. (See Figure 5.4.)

So the basis for the cumbersome DSM IIIR classification listed above is now explained. The patient suffering from a generalized anxiety state may avoid situations where he feels his already critical sense of insecurity is raised above the tolerable level ('agoraphobia without history of panic disorder'); the patient may have panic disorder but avoidance responses have not yet developed or the personality structure is robust enough to enable the patient to resist their development ('panic disorder without agoraphobia'); or the patient has continuing panic attacks and has developed the avoidance responses ('panic disorder with agoraphobia'). The DSM IIIR classification is in fact incomplete since it omits the state of agoraphobic-type fears preceded by panic disorder but in which the disorder is now quiescent (agoraphobia with history of panic disorder). This is important and a source of incorrect management; patients will often continue to refer to their anxiety on approaching their feared locations as 'panic attacks' but these are of a different quality to the original attacks. The biogenic panic disorder may respond to antidepressant medication but the situationally determined anxiety will not respond to drug treatment and will respond to psychological therapy (see Chapter 7).

Although Freud recognized and described a panic attack, the interest in panic disorder and its classification as a separate form of anxiety has only occurred since an American psychiatrist, D. F. Klein in 1964, recognized that panic disorder did not improve with the prescription of sedative drugs but did respond to the antidepressant drug imipramine. Subsequent studies have shown a response to other drugs marketed as antidepressants, including monoamine oxidase inhibitors, but if the disorder is basically a biogenic (endogenous) form of mood disorder the underlying neurochemical mechanism has not been reliably confirmed (see Chapter 3), nor any explanation forthcoming as to what precipitates the first attack. A clinical psychologist, David Clark in Oxford, has

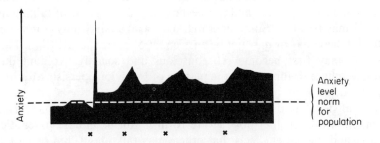

Figure 5.4: Panic attack occurring in situation (**x**) with subsequent anxiety when situation is again approached

attempted a different explanation for the disorder. He proposes that the panic attacks result from catastrophic misinterpretations of certain bodily sensations, mainly those which are involved in normal anxiety responses such as palpitations, breathlessness or dizziness; experiencing such sensations the individual then becomes alarmed that he is suffering from a serious illness and anxiety spirals upwards increasing the underlying bodily discomfort, which in turn adds further fuel to the mounting anxiety until a state of panic is reached. This 'cognitive theory' of the disorder denies any primary 'endogenous' disturbance of mood and asserts that, even when no obvious anxiety precedes the full-blown attack, there is always some quite innocuous event such as suddenly getting up from the sitting position (dizziness), exercise (breathlessness, palpitations) or drinking coffee (palpitations) which triggers the attack. There is also a weakness in this theory for it does not explain why the person should experience such overwhelming terror on a particular occasion when he must have experienced such somatic disturbances on countless occasions in the past with no more than the usual mild discomfort. The disorder awaits a comprehensive explanation.

Social Anxiety

Of all situations which create anxiety, the commonest are those involving social interaction or simply being observed by other people. The common fears of the agoraphobic type involve predicaments where the person is trapped in a situation from which he cannot easily escape without becoming the object of curiosity or contempt; such situations are standing in queues or sitting in a row with other people in a public building such as a theatre.

Social anxiety is a consequence of feelings of insecurity and sensitivity to the remarks of others. It usually commences in childhood and becomes entrenched, for, no matter how many successful interactions the person may have with others, he broods about those he regards as his failures. The tendency of children to band together in groups to tease or mock the child who appears in any way unusual is a major cause of social anxiety. The child who forgets his piece when called upon to stand before the class and recite may sense the amused titters of the other children, approaches the situation again with dread, is then more likely to make some error, and the seed of an enduring fear of talking in front of others may be sown. Sometimes marked social anxiety may commence later in life and there may or may not be an account of some specific triggering event. A person may first become self-conscious and socially avoidant during a depressive phase or illness and the pattern of behaviour persists after recovery from the depression.

Social anxiety based upon low self-confidence may pervade many aspects of the patient's life. In the most severe form it can be almost psychotic in its intensity and the patient feels that others may talk about him or look at him in a meaningful way (ideas of reference); he becomes more and more isolated and averse to any contact with people, ending up as an anchorite. In other cases social anxiety is focused upon a specific type of interaction, for example being interviewed, eating in the company of others, the fear of blushing, trembling or passing urine in a public urinal. The list of possible social anxieties is, of course, endless.

Illness Anxiety (Hypochondriasis)

Ranking not far below social anxieties in terms of frequency are those people who are beset by anxiety in relation to their own health or the health of others. Anxiety in this area may be classified in several ways, but the classification followed here will be:

1 Phobia of illness
2 Fear of the actual presence of illness
3 Anxiety-complicating physical illness
4 Disease-claiming behaviour

Phobia of illness usually focuses on one particular theme such as seeing people vomit, physical deformity, cancer or AIDS. The sufferer may be able to trace back the origin of the phobia to a specific incident occurring perhaps many years previously and the anxiety, as is the case with isolated phobias, may be very specific. For instance, a woman was unable to join in the village gossip in case she heard the word cancer; she even avoided reading newspapers in case she came across the word. Her thoughts flew to the possibility of the disease if she, or any member of her family, had the slightest pain the cause of which was not immediately obvious, such as her own attacks of migraine. She was 44 years old and the condition had been present for 20 years since her mother died from cancer of the breast. She herself was prone to seasonal episodes of depression and she recollected that she was suffering from depression at the time she learned of her mother's diagnosis.

Fear of a physical illness which eludes the physician's diagnostic skill is frequently based upon the presence of one of the somatic symptoms of tension, usually muscular pain. The failure to detect the presence of an anxiety state frequently leads to a patient being subjected to repeated physical examination in different hospital departments, numbers of inconclusive investigations and a variety of ineffective treatments. All these procedures enhance the concern about the elusive 'disease' and worry serves to aggravate and prolong the symptoms. This iatrogenic disorder represents an enormous burden of human suffering and health service expenditure. The early use of the simple self-assessment Hospital Anxiety and Depression (HAD) Scale (see Chapter 6) will give the lead to the basis of the symptoms and correct management in a large proportion of these patients.

Actual physical illness may be aggravated by anxiety. The very discomfort of the symptoms and possibly the sinister, life-threatening nature of the illness will cause anxiety which will in turn intensify the suffering and complicate the management. In some cases anxiety complicating illness may worsen the prognosis, as for instance when anxiety about the presence of hypertension leads to a sustained or episodic increase of the blood pressure. Enquiry about the presence of anxiety, perhaps supplemented by an HAD Scale rating, should be a part of every medical examination.

Finally there is that difficult group of patients for whom attendance at hospitals and general practitioners' surgeries has become a way of life. The most florid cases are labelled as suffering from the Munchausen syndrome but a more general term — the hospital addiction syndrome — has now been substituted. A better term for the less florid case is 'disease-claiming behaviour'. These patients must be distinguished from the other groups described above. They have the appearance of great concern about whatever symptoms they present and manipulate their doctors into ever more referrals, usually changing to another practitioner when one calls a halt to referrals and 'treatments'. They may have the outward appearance of anxiety and concern but in fact derive true satisfaction from the physicians' concern, bafflement and ineffective efforts to treat them. They invariably become extremely angry when challenged with the true state of affairs.

Sexual Anxiety

Anxiety focused upon sexual function, what Masters and Johnson termed 'performance anxiety', is the basis of most sexual dysfunction; this term refers to difficulty in sexual intercourse in a heterosexual relationship, i.e. the group of disorders which used to be termed impotence and frigidity but for which more exact terms are now used in professional communications. The disorders are those of sexual arousal: general sexual dysfunction; disorders of the vasocongestive phase: erectile dysfunction in the male; disorders of the orgasmic phase: anorgasmia (female) and premature ejaculation or inability to ejaculate (male). The condition of vaginismus in women is not easily classified into one or other of the phases of the sexual response.

Anxiety is, of course, not the sole cause of sexual dysfunction. Important factors to be taken into account in the assessment of a couple presenting with a sexual problem are the quality of their relationship; the basic sexual orientation of each partner (concealed, but unadmitted homosexual preference may be the cause of an aversion to a sexual relationship); physical illness; and drugs or alcohol. A loss of sexual arousal occurring in the setting of a relationship in which sexual intercourse was previously enjoyed may be the presenting feature of a low-grade depressive illness requiring antidepressant drug treatment not conjoint marital counselling. When these various factors have been considered and excluded, performance anxiety remains. Anxiety about sexual capacity will invariably inhibit the performance and psychosexual therapy must be based upon techniques to overcome anxiety and regain self-esteem.

Simple Phobic State

Apart from the themes of social interaction, illness and going away from home or travelling considered above, anxiety may focus on a wide range of objects or situations. Among the commonest are spiders, moths, worms and snakes, cats, dogs, thunderstorms, gales, aeroplanes and closed-in spaces such as lifts. The severely phobic patient will take considerable precautions to avoid contact with his feared situation; for instance, the storm phobic will seek complete assurance from weather forecasters and barometers before going out of his home. There is frequently a confusion about the difference between a phobia and an obsession. The obsessional patient fears not so much the object itself as the possible consequences of contact with the object. Thus a person with a phobia of dogs will experience extreme fear at the sight of a dog; the obsessional will not experience so much fear in the presence of the dog but will feel compelled to engage in prolonged rituals of cleaning after the dog has departed in case it has left behind some contamination. The obsessional feels compelled to carry out rituals or ruminative thoughts to ward off 'danger' which he knows to be non-existent.

The cause of phobic states is debatable. Freud and his followers hold them to be mental devices by which danger is externalized and which thereby serve to ward off a hidden internal danger. This view has been largely replaced, in the wake of behaviourism, by simple association of anxiety with the object that comes to be feared, for example the patient, as a child, found a large spider among her cornflakes, became extremely distraught and thereafter avoidance of spiders strengthens the fear and leads to its perpetuation. Such a theory is, of course, simplistic, especially since the supposed psychotraumatic initial acquaintance with the object cannot always be traced. Many phobic patients are prone to depressive episodes and frequently the onset of the phobia occurs during such an episode and the phobia remains as a permanent feature after the depression remits. The same phenomenon is seen in obsessionals and it seems as if the state of depression provides fertile emotional soil in which the seed of the fear may germinate. Once established, phobias persist; they do not wax and wane in intensity or undergo periods of remission. There is usually no other psychiatric abnormality nor does any one personality type predominate.

Childhood Anxiety

As in adults, anxiety in children may be generalized or focus upon specific objects or situations. The characteristic episodic anxiety of the panic disorder syndrome occurs also in children, although it is more likely to be misdiagnosed as a disorder of behaviour. The anxiety state may occur in the setting of familial emotional disturbance or it may follow some such upsetting experience as a bereavement or admission to hospital. In early childhood phobias commonly centre on the themes of animals, the dark, noise and illness or death. As soon as the child starts to attend school, the school may become the focus of anxiety. Some children have marked separation anxiety from an early age and the early weeks at the first school cause emotional storms and upheaval.

The so-called 'school phobia' or 'school refusal' may commence at a later age in a child who has had no major difficulty in adapting to the earlier experience of separation from the home. The condition affects boys and girls equally and may commence gradually or suddenly although an acute onset is commoner in younger children. In older children there is a more gradual onset occurring in the setting of a withdrawal from peer group activities. There may be a preceding experience which appears to be related to the onset of the disorder such as a death in the family or move to a new school but such precipitants are not invariable. The child may allow himself to be taken to school but then run home again or set off to school on his own and only get halfway there before turning back. A high level of generalized anxiety may be present and this is likely to manifest as somatic symptoms. Depressive disorder in the parents is common.

John, aged 10, had recently moved to a new school when he developed severe anxiety about attendance at school. His parents were aware that his distress was real and requested a medical opinion; they wisely stopped trying to push him to attend school pending expert advice on management. He had previous mild trait anxiety which caused little concern and was mainly manifest as shyness. Following the onset of the school refusal he began to sleep badly and his appetite diminished so that he lost weight; he complained of abdominal pain which was always worse on any morning when there was a need to leave home and meet new people. His older sister had had a similar problem and his father had suffered from a depressive disorder although he had recovered before the onset of John's anxiety.

Anxiety as Symptom of Other Mental Disorder

Anxiety may be symptomatic of other psychiatric disorders, especially those in which the whole structure of personal integrity becomes threatened in some way which appears inexplicable to the patient. However, the relationship of anxiety to depressive states provides the most important diagnostic challenge and is the source of the greatest errors in treatment. In order to clarify thinking it is vital to determine, by careful examination, in just what sense the term 'depression' is being used in any individual patient. It was noted, soon after the introduction of the first effective antidepressant drugs, the monoamine oxidase inhibitors, that some 'anxiety states' responded to their prescription and so the term 'atypical depression' was proposed. This phenomenon has been confirmed by subsequent clinical practice and other antidepressant drugs have been shown to be effective. The question therefore arises as to which anxiety states may be expected to respond to such treatment? The patient suffering from an incapacitating anxiety state may become 'depressed' in the sense of being demoralized; he may also have, or develop, a poor self-image, low self-esteem. In neither of these two senses of the ubiquitous term 'depression' would a response to antidepressant drug treatment be predicted. The mood of sadness is too universal to be a guide to treatment response; disturbances of appetite and sleep likewise do not discriminate and suicidal ideation occurs only in the more severe states. The best symptomatic marker of an underlying biogenic depressive disorder is the state of anhedonia, the pervasive loss of the ability to experience pleasure in any circumstance. Anhedonia is a quiet state, not revealed unless specific enquiry is made, and may be quite overshadowed by the more flamboyant symptoms of anxiety; but if, on careful enquiry, the patient has lost enjoyment in all previously enjoyed occupations and relationships, if he has lost enjoyment of food, of sexual pleasure and his sense of humour, if he no longer responds to some normally pleasurable experience such as music or flowers, and if this state is persistent, then the anhedonic depressive state is confirmed. The HAD Scale, the depression subscale of which is based upon the anhedonic state, will reveal a high depression as well as a high anxiety score. In this state psychotherapeutic intervention is likely to be ineffective and an antidepressant drug should be prescribed.

FURTHER READING

Clark, D. M. A cognitive approach to panic. *Behav Ther Res* 1986; **24**: 461–470.
Klein, D. F. Differentiation of two drug-responsive anxiety syndromes. *Psycho Pharmacol* 1964; **5**: 397–408.
Tyrer, P. *The Role of Bodily Feelings in Anxiety*. Oxford: Oxford University Press, 1976.

Chapter 6

Assessment for Treatment

So far we have considered the different aspects of anxiety, the different senses in which the word is used, anxiety as a normal state and the different manifestations of morbid anxiety. In so far as anxiety is a normal aspect of life, most anxious people do not consider themselves to be in need of professional help. However, the role of anxiety in the wide range of distress from stammering to back pain, from phobia of dental treatment to insomnia, is being increasingly defined and with definition comes consideration of treatment. The enormous number of prescriptions for sedative drugs is evidence of the readiness to diagnose anxiety at the root of the distress; it has been estimated that in Britain one person in every five takes a benzodiazepine drug at some time and one person in every twenty takes such a drug regularly.

The advice as regards need for treatment must rest upon a careful assessment of the person, his circumstances, his distress or symptoms and his motivation for change and attitude to treatment. The person must be enabled to give his own account of his distress but there should be a structure to the interview and he should be guided from one area to the next, so that at the end of the interview a provisional understanding of the person, his background and his distress has emerged. An interview with an informant who knows the person well is usually helpful and permission may be sought for this. In the case of a young child the account is probably given by a parent and in this situation the interviewer must covertly assess the parent and the family relationships as well as the child, for an emotionally disturbed mother is more likely to report abnormality in her child.

Information should be acquired about the following aspects of the person and his relationships:

- The complaint or symptom, its duration and course
- Other symptoms of emotional distress or psychiatric disorder
- To what, if anything, does the person attribute his distress?
- The present circumstances and stress including personal relationships and support or the lack of it
- Present physical health. The consumption of drugs and alcohol and whether these have recently changed in quantity

70

- The basic personality structure, especially in respect to trait anxiety. How effectively the person may have coped with stress in the past
- If anxiety is established as the basis of the current distress, how ready is the person to accept a psychological explanation?
- Motivation for change and acceptance of treatment plan

THE COMPLAINT

The likelihood that the complaint is a manifestation of anxiety is assessed in terms of the knowledge of the psychopathology of anxiety and the relationship of the complaint to stress at present and in the past. The basic symptomatology of an anxiety state was covered in Chapter 5. A useful assessment procedure of the presence and overall severity of morbid anxiety is the Clinical Anxiety Scale (CAS). This was developed from the widely used Hamilton Anxiety Scale but has certain advantages over the latter instrument. It is briefer (just six items); the large number of items relating to somatic symptomatology have been removed so that the CAS is valid when used in the setting of physical illness; there are clear instructions for allotting grades to the items; the CAS is designed to assess the present state of anxiety over the past week or so and not just the severity in the interview situation; score ranges are provided which enable the interpretation of the score in terms of clinically meaningful categories— absent, mild, moderate and severe. The Clinical Anxiety Scale is presented in Appendix 6.1.

Completion of the Clinical Anxiety Scale will take about 10 minutes of the interviewer's time. Another useful assessment device, completed by the patient in three or four minutes, is the Hospital Anxiety and Depression (HAD) Scale— see Appendix 6.1. This instrument was developed for use in general hospital medical and surgical departments and, like the CAS, avoids emphasis on somatic symptoms or disturbances such as of appetite or sleep which may equally be symptomatic of physical as of emotional disorder. It has the further advantages of distinguishing anxiety from the largely biogenic (anhedonic) depressive state and presenting the range of scores for each construct in terms of normal, borderline and morbid. The word 'hospital' in the title of the HAD Scale does not imply that it is invalid for use in primary care or community settings.

Both the CAS and HAD Scale give information on the presence and severity of generalized, or pervasive, anxiety. However, an anxiety-based complaint may be focused specifically on some area and the level of generalized anxiety may be within the normal range. It is therefore useful to supplement the interview with a further self-assessment device, taking a few minutes to complete, which picks out anxiety focused on special situations such as travelling, being observed by others and illness. This Focused Anxiety Schedule is also reproduced in Appendix 6.1.

It is necessary to establish how the complaint commenced, whether suddenly or gradually, whether in the setting of some other illness or psychiatric disorder and whether at a time of emotional stress or in relationship to some specific psychotraumatic incident. Since the onset, has the complaint waxed and waned in intensity or have there been periods when it has been absent only to return? In the case of women it is important to enquire whether the symptom changes in relation to the phase of the menstrual cycle; if it is characteristically present only in the days before menstruation or much worse at the time then consideration may be given to the need for hormone (progesterone) replacement therapy. Before deciding on this issue it is helpful to request the woman to keep a 'diary' of the complaint in relationship to menstruation and an acceptable chart for this use is shown in Appendix 6.1.

PERSONALITY, BACKGROUND AND PRESENT LIFESTYLE

The interviewer should now seek to develop an understanding of the person in depth. It is helpful to say why this information is required and to gain the person's cooperation with the interview when it turns towards more personal matters. There should be no fixed set of questions but the interview should lead to some knowledge of: what sort of person is this? what sort of life has he led? what sort of life is he leading now?

Personality traits are of infinite variety and it is not possible to go through them all. In the case of investigation of a complaint which is probably based upon anxiety, the important traits are: proneness to anxiety, rigidity, dependence, sensitivity and perfectionism. Proneness to anxiety is assessed in terms of habitual tendency to worry excessively and habitual overarousal indicated by poor sleep and difficulty in relaxing; in fact all the 'state' items of the Clinical Anxiety Scale may be adapted to trait items to assess the personality structure. Rigidity of personality is assessed in terms of the difficulty in adapting to change and dealing with circumstances which upset routine. Sensitivity refers to the habitual tendency to fear that one's performance will be judged adversely by others and this may be linked to an exaggerated response to criticism or what is perceived as criticism. Perfectionism is an exaggerated concern about one's standards of achievement in some respect or other, with consequent unnecessary self-criticism when it is felt that the standard has not been achieved.

The person's background cannot be understood in any depth except in long-term psychodynamic therapy, and even then the account will be highly influenced by selective recall and distortion. However, it is necessary to know whether the person's experience of vicissitudes may have been beyond the normal and, if so, how he coped and what sort of enduring features resulted, for example a chronic sense of insecurity from unstable home background. It is equally important to know whether the person has led a life free from major stress so that any present adversity is a new experience for which he is ill prepared to cope.

Present Circumstances

The present circumstances include not only an account of present stress but relationships with others, the support structure. Are there others with whom he can talk over his problems or discuss his complaint and, if so, are their attitudes helpful or the reverse? Does the person have sufficient occupation and diversion or are his days passed in a manner which seems to him to be empty and boring? This is the natural stage of the interview at which to raise the topic of alcohol consumption and whether this has recently changed or whether it is at a level where problems may result or have resulted. The use of drugs, prescribed and purchased, should also be established and, again, whether there has been any change in the dose or pattern of consumption.

A useful device which enables the interviewer to understand the present lifestyle is to ask the person to provide an account of a typical day in his life, from getting up to going to bed again.

PHYSICAL AND MENTAL HEALTH

Enquiry must be made about this in the past and present. Some anxiety-based symptoms may be understood to have originated in the setting of physical ill-health and sometimes worry about health leads to their perpetuation. Some somatic symptoms of anxiety, especially pain, are so similar to physical symptoms that the person cannot be convinced of their psychogenic nature until he has received an adequate physical examination; however, once there is no doubt in the mind of the physician that there is no physical basis for the symptom, then the person should be fully informed and further referrals for examinations and investigations should cease.

Adequate knowledge of the past mental health and of the constitutional proneness to psychiatric disorder, as indicated by a marked familial history, may clarify some apparently obscure disorders. Anxiety may mask depressive illness and persist once a depressive illness has remitted (see Chapter 5).

ATTITUDE TO THE COMPLAINT
AND MOTIVATION TO CHANGE

Once the conclusion has been reached that the distress or symptoms presented by the patient are a manifestation of anxiety, the patient must be given an explanation including a summary of the past and present factors that have combined to result in the distress. Time should be allowed for reflection and perhaps, at the next session, the patient should be asked to give his view of any significant aspects which the explanation failed to take into account and whether the explanation makes reasonable sense. Management of anxiety by whatever reassurance or treatment plan will not progress far unless the anxiety basis of the distress is accepted. Further time may be required to review the evidence for diagnosis but this time will be less than the time wasted in pursuing treatment which the patient does not accept as appropriate for his condition. If the HAD or Clinical Anxiety Scale has been completed by this stage, information as to how he scored may be helpful but, of course, anxiety may be channelled into a single symptom or situation without any generalized anxiety being present.

Most difficulty is experienced in those cases where anxiety is biogenic, is experienced as a panic attack with severe somatic symptoms and no apparent cause to account for the attack. Such attacks may, rarely, occur in the setting of organic brain disorder (see Chapter 3) and the intensity of the experience is sufficient to cause the sufferer to doubt that the distress is 'just anxiety'. In such cases time must be spent in reviewing what is known about the panic disorder syndrome.

Treatment need not be prescribed at the first interview. Indeed, it is usually better to point out that anxiety sometimes serves a purpose of focusing attention on problems and thereby working towards solutions. The availability or otherwise of the various therapeutic procedures such as counselling and psychological management should be discussed and if a pharmacological treatment is to be offered the benefit and risks of such prescription should be understood. Sedative drugs must never be prescribed without underlining the risk of dependence or their potentiation of the effect of alcohol.

The overall motivation for change should be gauged, especially if this requires cooperation and consistent application to a psychological treatment programme where the main benefit must rest on what the person does to help himself to overcome anxiety. Usually it is advisable to provide a simple written explanation of the mode of the therapy and to advise the person to make his own decision whether or not he will commit himself to it.

Appendix 6.1:

Assessment Scales

Clinical Anxiety Scale
Instructions for Use

The Scale is an instrument for the assessment of the present state of anxiety; therefore the emphasis on eliciting information for the ratings should be on how the patient feels at the present time. However, the interview itself may raise, or lower, the severity of anxiety and the interviewer should inform the patient that he should describe how he has felt during the period of the past two days.

Psychic tension

(care should be taken to distinguish tension from muscular tension — see next item)

Score 4: Very marked and distressing feeling of being 'on edge', 'keyed up', 'wound up', or 'nervous' which persists with little change throughout the waking hours.

Score 3: As above, but with some fluctuation of severity during the course of the day.

Score 2: A definite experience of being tense which is sufficient to cause some, although not severe, distress.

Score 1: A slight feeling of being tense which does not cause distress.

Score 0: No feeling of being tense apart from the normal degree of tension experienced in response to stress and which is acceptable as normal for the population.

Ability to relax

(muscular tension)

Score 4: The experience of severe tension throughout much of the bodily musculature which may be accompanied by such symptoms as pain, stiffness, spasmodic contractions, and lack of control over movements. The experience is present throughout most of the waking day and there is no ability to produce relaxation at will.

Score 3: As above, but the muscular tension may only be experienced in certain groups of muscles and may fluctuate in severity throughout the day.

Score 2: A definite experience of muscular tension in some part of the musculature sufficient to cause some, but not severe, distress.

Score 1: Slight recurrent muscular tension of which the patient is aware but which does not cause distress. Very mild degrees of tension headache or pain in other groups of muscles should be scored here.

Score 0: No subjective muscular tension or of such degree which, when it occurs, can easily be controlled at will.

Startle response

(hyperarousability)

Score 4: Unexpected noise causes severe distress so that the patient may complain in some such phrase as 'I jump out of my skin'. Distress is experienced in psychic *and* somatic modalities so that, in addition to the experience of fright, there is muscular activity and autonomic symptoms such as sweating or palpitation.

Score 3: Unexpected noise causes severe distress in psychic or somatic, but not in both modalities.

Score 2: Unexpected noise causes definite but not severe distress.

Score 1: The patient agrees that he is slightly 'jumpy' but is not distressed by this.

Score 0: The degree of startle response is entirely acceptable as normal for the population.

Worrying

(the assessment must take into account the degree to which worry is out of proportion to actual stress)

Score 4: The patient experiences almost continuous preoccupation with painful thoughts which cannot be stopped voluntarily and the distress is quite out of proportion to the subject matter of the thoughts.

Score 3: As above, but there is some fluctuation in intensity throughout the waking hours and the distressing thoughts may cease for an hour or two, especially if the patient is distracted by activity requiring his attention.

Score 2: Painful thoughts out of proportion to the patient's situation keep intruding into consciousness but he is able to dispel or dismiss them.

Score 1: The patient agrees that he tends to worry a little more than necessary about minor matters but this does not cause much distress.

Score 0: The tendency to worry is accepted as being normal for the population; for instance even marked worrying over a severe financial crisis or unexpected illness in a relative should be scored as 0 if it is judged to be entirely in keeping with the degree of stress.

Apprehension

Score 4: The experience is that of being on the brink of some disaster which cannot be explained. The experience need not be continuous and may occur in short bursts several times a day.

Score 3: As above, but the experience does not occur more than once a day.

Score 2: A sensation of groundless apprehension of disaster which is not severe although it causes definite distress. The patient may not use strong terms such as 'disaster' or 'catastrophe' but may express his experience in some such phrase as 'I feel as if something bad is about to happen'.

Score 1: A slight degree of apprehensiveness of which the patient is aware but which does not cause distress.

Score 0: No experience of groundless anticipation of disaster.

Restlessness

Score 4: The patient is unable to keep still for more than a few minutes and engages in restless pacing or other purposeless activity.

Score 3: As above, but he is able to keep still for an hour or so at a time.

Score 2: There is a feeling of 'needing to be on the move' which causes some, but not severe, distress.

Score 1: Slight experience of restlessness which causes no distress.

Score 0: Absence of restlessness.

GRADE	RECOVERED	MILD	MODERATE	SEVERE
RANGE	0 – 4	5 – 10	11 – 16	17 – 24

Reproduced from *British Journal of Psychiatry* 1982; **141**: 518–23; 1986; **148**: 599–601.

The Hospital Anxiety and Depression (HAD) Scale

Name: Date:

Doctors are aware that emotions play an important part in most illnesses. If your doctor knows about these feelings will be able to help you more.

This questionnaire is designed to help your doctor to know how you feel. Ignore the numbers printed on the le of the questionnaire. Read each item and underline the reply which comes closest to how you have been feeling the past week.

Don't take too long over your replies; your immediate reaction to each item will probably be more accurate than long thought out response.

	A			D		
		I feel tense or 'wound up'				**I feel as if I am slowed down**
	3	Most of the time		3		Nearly all the time
	2	A lot of the time		2		Very often
	1	From time to time, occasionally		1		Sometimes
	0	Not at all		0		Not at all
D		**I still enjoy the things I used to enjoy**			A	**I get a sort of frightened feeling like 'butterflies**
0		Definitely as much				**in the stomach**
1		Not quite so much			0	Not at all
2		Only a little			1	Occasionally
3		Hardly at all			2	Quite often
					3	Very often
	A	**I get a sort of frightened feeling as if something**				
		awful is about to happen				**I have lost interest in my appearance**
	3	Very definitely and quite badly		D		Definitely
	2	Yes, but not too badly		3		I don't take so much care as I should
	1	A little, but it doesn't worry me		2		I may not take quite as much care
	0	Not at all		1		I take just as much care as ever
				0		
D		**I can laugh and see the funny side of things**			A	**I feel restless as if I have to be on the move**
0		As much as I always could			3	Very much indeed
1		Not quite so much now			2	Quite a lot
2		Definitely not so much now			1	Not very much
3		Not at all			0	Not at all
	A	**Worrying thoughts go through my mind**				**I look forward with enjoyment to things**
	3	A great deal of the time		D		As much as ever I did
	2	A lot of the time		0		Rather less than I used to
	1	From time to time but not too often		1		Definitely less than I used to
	0	Only occasionally		2		Hardly at all
				3		
D		**I feel cheerful**			A	**I get sudden feelings of panic**
3		Not at all			3	Very often indeed
2		Not often			2	Quite often
1		Sometimes			1	Not very often
0		Most of the time			0	Not at all
	A	**I can sit at ease and feel relaxed**				**I can enjoy a good book or radio or TV programme**
	0	Definitely		D		Often
	1	Usually		0		Sometimes
	2	Not often		1		Not often
	3	Not at all		2		Very seldom
				3		

Now check you have answered all questions

FOR HOSPITAL USE ONLY
D (8–10)
A (8–10)

(After Zigmond and Snaith, 1983. *Acta Psychiatrica Scandinavica* **67**: 361–70.)

The Focused Anxiety Schedule

NAME............................. DATE............

Here is a list of situations in which people sometimes feel unduly anxious.

0 = No anxiety   1 = Mild anxiety   2 = Very anxious

Check through the list and if you feel anxiety at the 1 or 2 level in any of the situations, make a pencil circle around the appropriate number.

0	1	2	Cats
0	1	2	Walking away from home
0	1	2	Thunderstorms
0	1	2	Being alone
0	1	2	Injections, hypodermic needles
0	1	2	Being watched by others
0	1	2	Spiders
0	1	2	Aches and pains
0	1	2	People in authority
0	1	2	Bus travel
0	1	2	Supermarkets
0	1	2	Snakes
0	1	2	People being sick, vomiting
0	1	2	Walking across empty spaces
0	1	2	High winds
0	1	2	Being in queues
0	1	2	Blood
0	1	2	The dark
0	1	2	Confined spaces, e.g. lifts
0	1	2	Eating in presence of others
0	1	2	Mice

If you have a fear of a particular situation not in this list, make a note of it here:

This scale may be reproduced providing full acknowledgement is made to source.

Menstrual Symptom Chart

Day	Month		Month		Month		Name:
		M		M		M	Year: 198
1		|		|		|	
2		|		|		|	M: Menstruating
3		|		|		|	
4		|		|		|	
5		|		|		|	
6		|		|		|	
7		|		|		|	+ ----------------
8		|		|		|	
9		|		|		|	
10		|		|		|	
11		|		|		|	
12		|		|		|	
13		|		|		|	
14		|		|		|	o ----------------
15		|		|		|	
16		|		|		|	
17		|		|		|	
18		|		|		|	
19		|		|		|	
20		|		|		|	// ----------------
21		|		|		|	
22		|		|		|	
23		|		|		|	
24		|		|		|	Use above symbols
25		|		|		|	to indicate symptoms
26		|		|		|	to be assessed in
27		|		|		|	relation to timing of
28		|		|		|	menstrual cycle
29		|		|		|	
30		|		|		|	
31		|		|		|	

Chapter 7

The Management of Anxiety

The effective management of anxiety must be based upon knowledge of the nature of disorders which present as states of anxiety, the interplay of biological and experiential factors that have resulted in the state and an understanding of the therapeutically active ingredients of the various treatment strategies. Frequently explanation, discussion and reassurance are sufficient to bring about improvement and sometimes the person can be advised how to bring about his own improvment rather than engaging upon treatment with a therapist. Sometimes, as discussed in preceding sections of this book, the anxiety is essentially biogenic and a drug treatment may be necessary but more often a psychological approach is to be advised. The choice of approach must depend upon the availability of workers with sufficient training to carry out the particular therapy. Chronic disabling anxiety is ubiquitous and if the problem were to be effectively tackled there could never be sufficient therapists; therefore there is need for the development of cost-effective self-help methods requiring little input of professional time.

Before considering the psychological approaches the role of drugs will be discussed.

PHARMACOTHERAPY OF ANXIETY

Three classes of drugs are considered for the management of anxiety: (a) the sedative–hypnotic drugs; (b) drugs producing β-adrenergic blockade, the beta blockers; (c) the antidepressant drugs.

The Sedative–Hypnotic Drugs

The benzodiazepine drugs are currently the most widely prescribed drugs for anxiety. The effect of these drugs on the GABA neurotransmitter system of the central nervous system has been considered in Chapter 3. The hope that benzodiazepines would provide a safe and effective antidote to anxiety has not been sustained although they continue to be widely prescribed. In fact it was always a forlorn hope to seek a pharmacological solution to psychogenic anxiety.

The expectation is now shattered by the revelation of the potential of these drugs for producing states of physical dependence and distress when withdrawal is attempted. The manifestations of benzodiazepine withdrawal are severe anxiety of a quality unlike that for which the drug was first prescribed, nausea and retching, paraesthesia and a sense of distortion of the body, oversensitivity to noise and light, hallucinations and, in the case of abrupt withdrawal in a person dependent on a high dose, epileptic fits. Prolonged states of depression may occur following withdrawal and some preparations such as lorazepam appear to cause more dependence than others. Some long-term takers can stop the drug with very little discomfort, whereas for others the distress may be so intense that continued prescription is the lesser evil. Sedative drugs cause somnolence which may put the person at risk and another risk is the increase of the effect of alcohol. States of depression and irritability may be made worse and will certainly not be relieved by a sedative drug. If they are prescribed at all it must be for very short periods of time and the person must be told of the risk of dependence.

Beta Blockers

Drugs that reduce the effect of stimulation of β-adrenergic receptor function may diminish the feedback of somatic sensation to the brain and the consequent increase of anxiety by awareness of the somatic consequences of anxiety. Stimulation of β-adrenergic receptors results in dilation of arteries and arterioles, increase in heart rate and cardiac output, dilation of the bronchi, renin release and increased glycogenolysis. Thus the main somatic manifestations of anxiety dependent on this function are flushing and palpitations. Beta blockers may reduce these effects but will have no effect on other major somatic manifestations of anxiety such as sweating, muscular spasms and tremor. The drugs will not reduce the consequences of hyperventilation and may indeed worsen asthma although selective blockers have been developed without effect on the bronchi. Beta blockers do not have much contribution to make to the therapy of anxiety but may be preferred by those who feel it imperative to prescribe, since they are free of the sedation and dependence-producing effects of the benzodiazepines.

Antidepressant Drugs

Anxiety, sometimes of overwhelming intensity, may mask a biogenic depressive state and in such cases the prescription of effective antidepressant drugs should not be delayed. Sedative drugs may worsen the depression and the tricyclic antidepressants have sufficient sedative effect; they have a long half-life, should usually be prescribed by a once daily dose and, if this is taken in the evening, severe insomnia, which is a constant feature of depression, will be relieved without the need for an additional hypnotic drug. Usually anxiety and depressive symptoms improve together, although sometimes anxiety may persist after depressive symptoms have abated.

The other anxiety state which responds to antidepressants is the biogenic panic disorder. A tricyclic antidepressant should be prescribed early in order to prevent the disabling consequences of repeated panic episodes. This is the case at any age, children included. However, a problem is the frequent intolerance of the drug, if it is prescribed in full dose, in the early stage of the treatment; sometimes there is a paradoxical increase of anxiety (see Chapter 3) and at other times sedation. In either case the effect is sufficient for many patients to refuse to continue the treatment and thereby lose the benefit of an effective remedy for what may become a protracted and disabling illness. The solution to this problem is prescription in very small dose in the first few days, gradually increasing the dose to a therapeutic level once the critical period for side-effects has passed: a dose of 25 mg of imipramine a day for the first week may then be increased up to 100 mg thereafter. Panic disorder responds to lower doses of anti-depressants than are required for depressive illness. Medication should be continued until the patient has been symptom-free for two or three months when it may be gradually reduced and stopped. The patient should be told that the disorder might reoccur and this would not constitute a failure of the treatment but would be an indication for its resumption. There is, so far, no evidence that any of the new non-tricyclic antidepressant drugs are either more effective in panic disorder or free from the problem of initial intolerance of side-effects.

No patient, of whatever age, should be denied effective pharmacotherapy and this calls for a closer alliance between psychotherapists and medically qualified doctors than exists. As previously described (Chapter 5), phobic states may arise in the setting of a depressive illness and the latter subsides to relieve the anxiety state as a permanent aftermath. In the absence of continuing depression there is no reason to prescribe antidepressants and psychological treatment may be commenced, but psychological treatment in the presence of a continuing biogenic disorder is not only ineffective but will increase the patient's demoralization on account of his failure to benefit from the treatment. The anhedonic state is the nearest clinical marker for a biogenic depressive state and this is recorded by the depression subscale of the HAD Scale. A chart of successive scores on the HAD may give the answer to some treatment failures. Figure 7.1 shows the

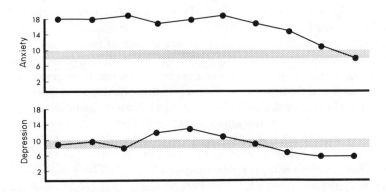

Figure 7.1: Hospital Anxiety and Depression Scale chart. Grey band indicates borderline between normal and abnormal scores

record of HAD scores in a patient who commenced a psychological anxiety management programme but did not make progress; the scores suggested that a depressive state was interfering with response to the therapy and examination revealed the presence of a mild but persistent and pervasive anhedonic state. Once this had been controlled by antidepressant drug treatment the psychotherapy led to improvement of the persisting anxiety.

ALCOHOL AND CAFFEINE

It is important to ask about the extent to which the patient attempts to alleviate anxiety by alcohol. Alcohol is certainly effective in reducing anxiety but reliance on this method is clearly a dangerous practice and many cases of alcoholic dependence commence in this way.

Excessive consumption of caffeinated beverages—coffee, tea and Coca-Cola—will induce a state of caffeinism; manifestations of this state are anxiety, restlessness and insomnia. Patients suffering from panic disorder may be especially sensitive to caffeine and a trial of decaffeinated beverages should be a preliminary to the institution of any other treatment procedure. Either by suggestion or by direct effect, the advice is sometimes successful.

THE TECHNIQUES OF PSYCHOTHERAPY

The systems of psychotherapy may be classified according to their basic premises about the nature of psychological disorder and the techniques for rectifying the disorders. The broad categories are: explorative therapies, behaviour therapies and cognitive therapies.

Explorative therapies are based upon the psychodynamic principle, that the disorder is to be understood in terms of the experiences of that person from birth onwards, especially his experience of personal relationships and the effect upon the developing psyche of particular stressful events. The techniques involve the retracing of this psychic development and, through this, the acquisition of self-knowledge and an understanding of the origins and nature of the disorder. Once the nature of the strange panics, obsessions or whatever else distress the person are comprehended they cease to alarm and so fade away.

The archetypal system of explorative therapy is Freudian psychoanalysis based upon the belief that infantile sexuality and the banishment from conscious recall of events surrounding this was at the root of neurotic disorder. The recall and unravelling of these psychotraumatic experiences might take several years and many hundreds of hours of therapist contact, and relief of distress was uncertain. Psychoanalysis was not the vehicle to bring relief to the great multitude who suffered from anxiety and other emotional disorder.

There followed extensive revisions and new ideas were supplied to enrich the variety of explorative therapies. The Freudian emphasis on infantile sexuality was soon jettisoned; Karen Horney, for instance, emphasized the importance of cultural factors and paid less attention to infantile events and more to the 'here and now' factors in the patient's ongoing experience. An important break with the analytic tradition occurred in the 1940s, when Carl Rogers in America discarded the belief that it was the analyst's insights and interpretations which healed the analysand. Rogers claimed that the function of the therapist was merely that of a sounding board, reflecting back to the client (Rogers did not use the word patient) the statements he had just uttered so that he might reflect upon these and the emotions which lay behind them, thus finding his own way through the maze of his psyche. The book of Rogerian therapy is called *Client Centred Therapy* and with it was launched the Encounter Movement and a great many of the concepts of the approaches collectively called counselling.

Behaviour therapy was launched in the late 1950s, when a South African psychiatrist, Joseph Wolpe, published his book *Psychotherapy by Reciprocal Inhibition*. Behaviourism is a branch of psychology dealing with the objective study of behaviour and the new therapy preached that behaviour such as phobic avoidance of situations could be directly modified in the here and now without any need to understand the individual's psychic development or the supposed factors determining the neurotic behaviour, be it phobia, compulsion, addiction, sexual deviation or whatever else. Wolpe in the Introduction to his book threw down the gauntlet to the dominant explorative therapies of the day: 'The ideal of medical treatment is to achieve the greatest effects in the shortest time. Today's most widely accepted regime for treatment of neurosis — psycho-analysis — is distinguished by the great length of the time it takes to produce results that are no better than those obtained by therapists using traditional methods customary in the psychiatric clinics of general hospitals'. Thus battle was joined, with the analysts predicting that behaviour therapy, based upon absurdly naive premises derived from observations in the animal laboratory, could at best only remove one symptom at the expense and substitution of some other symptom since the underlying fissures in the psyche had been left unhealed. However, the behaviour therapists were unshaken by such arguments and continued to treat phobias symptomatically by exposing their patients to the phobic situations and demonstrating that by one means or another they could overcome this fear. Under the influence of prestigious people such as Professor Hans Eysenck in Britain, clinical psychologists joined the small band of psychiatrists who were enthusiastic about the new approach and brought with them more objective methods of clinical experiment and outcome evaluation. It was shown that relief could be produced in weeks, not years, and that substitute symptoms apparently did not occur. The therapy was practicable in the state-funded health care systems of the world.

The 1970s saw the growth of therapeutic systems which are also based in the 'here and now' approach and which to a large extent developed out of the behavioural therapies. It was realized that the success of the latter occurred even although the individual was treated as if he were a laboratory rat and the therapist ignored the person's attitudes, expectations, beliefs and other aspects of the complex human psyche. Behaviour therapy was reinterpreted as a modification of the attitudes the person held about himself and his potential for self-mastery. Albert Ellis in his book *Reason and Emotion in Psychotherapy* quoted the first-century stoic philosopher Epictetus: 'Men are disturbed not by things but by the views they take of them'. The new therapies, which set out simply to reshape the person's destructive attitudes about himself, his low self-regard and prediction of failure, were the cognitive (or 'beliefs and attitudes') therapies. The apostles of this new approach, such as Professor Aaron Beck in America, have chosen to ignore all facets of human experience and psychological disorder which do not fit in with their chosen theory. For instance, 'depression' is overinterpreted as a disorder of attitudes, to the neglect of the biophysical abnormalities that manifest as mild depressive states. Nonetheless the cognitive therapies, selectively used, have added to the increasing variety of brief, effective interventions for emotional disorders and in particular for anxiety.

THE COMMON THERAPEUTIC FACTORS

The overwhelming tendency of psychotherapists of all persuasions is to become intensely absorbed in the theoretical structures they have elaborated or adopted, often ignoring contrary evidence to a ludicrous extent. A more profitable study now is not the attention to details of these contradicting theoretical systems but the study of the therapeutic factors common to all of them: what, in the process of therapy—no matter of what pretension to knowledge of psychological disorder—brings about improvement? An American observer of the psychotherapeutic scene, Jerome Frank, has made a study of these therapeutic factors which may be found, in varying amalgam and emphasis, in all therapies from Janov's primal scream to Jung's analytic psychology. They are:

1 An intense, emotionally charged confiding relationship with a helping person, often with the participation of a group
2 A rationale, or myth, which includes an explanation of the cause of the patient's distress and a method of relieving it. To be effective, the therapeutic myth must be compatible with the cultural world view by the patient and the therapist
3 Provision of new information concerning the nature and sources of the patient's problems and possible alternative ways of dealing with them
4 Strengthening of the patient's expectations of help through the personal qualities of the therapist, enhanced by his status in society and the setting in which he works
5 Provision of success experiences which further heighten the patient's hopes and also enhance his sense of mastery, interpersonal competence or capability, to mention some commonly used terms
6 The facilitation of emotional arousal which seems to be a prerequisite to attitudinal and behavioural change

In the evaluation of *Therapeutic Factors In Group Psychotherapy*, Sidney Bloch and Eric Crouch identified the following factors, which both confirm and expand Frank's common therapeutic factors:

1 Insight (self-understanding)
2 Learning from interpersonal action (interaction)
3 Acceptance (cohesiveness); the feeling of belonging to and support from the group
4 Self-disclosure, the divulging of intimate personal information
5 Catharsis: emotional release bringing some measure of relief
6 Guidance: the imparting of information and the giving of direct advice— either by the therapist or by the group
7 Universality: the realization that others share the same problems or symptoms
8 Altruism: benefit from extending help to others
9 Vicarious learning: change through the observation and perhaps imitation of others
10 The instillation of hope: the dawning of optimism through observation of change in others and oneself

All these factors, in one way or another and to a greater or a lesser extent, enter into the process of relief of distress by psychological therapies. In any particular approach or technique and with any particular patient we may speculate on which of the factors are operating and a greater benefit may be produced by enhancing the factor than by rigid adherence to the therapeutic technique. It may also then be understood that procedures which are not technically labelled as 'therapy' are in fact therapeutic and may be recommended, an example being the joining of a voluntary service organization to bring about one's own relief by helping others. Underpinning success with all approaches will be Frank's first and second factors: trust in the therapist and a faith in and understanding of the method.

One may challenge the statement that the relationship of the therapist with the patient or subject must be intense and 'emotionally charged'; one may also suspect that Rogers' prerequisite of an 'unconditional positive regard' of the therapist for his client may be overstated. The key term is perhaps confidence, the trust of the person in the competence of the therapist; a deeply emotional relationship is more likely to be antitherapeutic, prejudicing detached objective evaluation of the person and his situation, and emotional relationships have a habit of going awry, and with that the collapse of trust and confidence. But there must be confidence, for on that are built the other factors of expectations of relief, the acceptance of new information about the nature of the distress and the knowledge that expression of emotion will be accepted and utilized in the therapy. The person must also accept what Frank teasingly termed the 'myth' of the therapy; does the procedure, as briefly outlined, make sense to him? For instance, it will be quite pointless, in attempting to lead the person through a behavioural therapeutic programme, if he perceives this as quite pointless and all the time wishes to be enabled to arrive at some emotional *modus vivendi* with an overcritical parent or aggravating spouse. For this reason we again return to the importance of allowing the person time, after reflection on the explanations given, to make a personal decision of commitment to the therapy that is offered to him. This principle also holds if the treatment offered is to be the prescription of a drug.

THE ELEMENTS OF ANXIETY MANAGEMENT

Brief anxiety management techniques, generally categorized as 'cognitive–behavioural' methods, are now successfully practised although still poorly researched, especially with regard to long-term outcome after contact with the therapist has ceased. They are all composed of a variable mixture of the following elements:

- Explanation and motivation for change
- Relaxation or meditation
- Exposure to anxiety
- Restructuring of attitudes
- Self-control

In some techniques the guidance and encouragement of the therapist is of central importance, others emphasize group cohesion and example and others would dispense with the human element and rely on written, tape-recorded or computerized instructions. With limited resources to help all those who would benefit from reduction and control of anxiety, the degree of therapist input and hence cost effectiveness is of central importance and will require even greater emphasis in future research.

Explanation and Motivation

The first stage in devising an anxiety management programme is explanation, ensuring the patient's motivation for change and acceptance of the technique on offer. The person must understand the role of anxiety in his disorder or problem; in many cases this may be obvious, in others such as some eating disorders less obvious and in others such as persisting somatic pain the underlying anxiety may be obscure and denied. A sound physical examination must precede those cases of somatized anxiety before either the therapist or the patient can feel confident in an approach through anxiety management. Motivation for change is important and the person should have a broad grasp of the principles and practice of the proposed therapy. Some people have achieved a *modus vivendi* with their anxiety and the contemplation of the tasks of a life freed of the handicap may seem too great a challenge. Others may seek a change in which no personal effort is required.

The attitude of relatives is important. Relatives will usually play a key role in support and encouragement and there are cases in which the relative does not wish to see the balance of the relationship disturbed by major change and increase of self-confidence in the patient; a relative may even covertly sabotage a therapeutic programme. The most obvious example is the role of a spouse in helping the partner to overcome a sexual dysfunction based upon performance anxiety. Whenever possible the important relative, parent or spouse, should be seen and their cooperation enlisted.

A useful device is the provision of a brief written account of the therapy, its principles, what may be expected and how soon. The patient, and relative, should be advised to read the guide and make up his own mind whether he wants help of the type described. Any attempt to impose treatment on an anxious person is simply to invite non-cooperation.

Relaxation and Meditation

A therapeutic system devised by Jacobsen was presented in 1938 under the title of *Progressive Relaxation*. The method is based upon a system of exercises in which the person becomes proficient in muscular relaxation through deliberate tension and then letting go; an excerpt is:

> 'Now the muscles of your forehead — the muscles you frown with — make them as tight as possible — frown as hard as you can — that's it tighter — and tighter, a deep furrow in the centre of your forehead — so tight that you long to release the tension — but you don't — tighter still, hold it — a moment or two longer before letting go — now let go — that's it — deep relaxation replacing tension — forehead muscles smooth — and relaxed — feeling relaxed . . .'

and so on. The development of self-mastery is the essence of this at first sight naive method. The person is shown how to do something for himself, to induce a bodily change and through it a state of mental calmness, through a regular self-disciplined system of exercises. Later the concept of cue-control relaxation was introduced, i.e. the person learns to induce immediate mental quietude through concentrating on a stimulus such as the picture of a flower which had been associated with the physical relaxation exercises. The mental imagery of the picture acts as a 'panic button' which the person can press in case of need. Success entails a sense of self-mastery over anxiety.

In the procedure of biofeedback the person learns to control some bodily function such as heart rate or muscle tension by concentrating on the sound of a tone which has been electronically produced by this bodily function. Through concentrating on lowering the pitch of the audible tone he is in fact exerting control over the bodily function and thereby discovering that he has mastery over the functions of his own body.

The term meditation is used here in the sense of a state of intense concentration upon some mental device such as an image, the repetitious words of a prayer or a bodily sensation to the exclusion of other thought and sensory distractions in the environment. Meditation is an integral feature of many religious practices, an account of which is given by Daniel Goleman in *The Varieties of The Meditative Experience.*

An American physician, Herbert Benson, searching for a therapeutic device to combat the distress of drug withdrawal states, looked for a neutral term to replace the word meditation and used the phrase 'the relaxation response'. He summarized the basic components of all meditational systems, therapeutic and religious, under the headings: (a) a mental device, (b) a passive attitude, (c) decreased muscle tonus, (d) a quiet environment. The mental device is an image, words or bodily sensation on which the meditator focuses his attention to the virtual exclusion of all else. The passive attitude is the frame of mind in which the meditator 'invites' the experience rather than actively strives to perceive it; the difference in emphasis with regard to muscular relaxation between Jacobsen's procedure and meditation may be emphasized — in the former the subject will concentrate on actively contracting muscles and then relaxing whereas in the latter the subject will allow his mind to engage on the concept 'relaxation coming all through me'. The change of emphasis is important, for in the former the mental activity will distract from the concept of mental quietude.

The trance state induced in hypnotism is a state of meditation in which the subject dissociates his attention from other thoughts and sensations to dwell upon some suggested theme. Traditionally, the practice of hypnosis both in the entertainment and the therapeutic setting has focused upon the concept of the hypnotist and not the subject as the active inducer of the trance state although James Braid, who introduced the term hypnotism, realized that it was the subject and not the therapist who induced the trance. Meditation greatly facilitates the effect of suggestion and autosuggestion, a fact appreciated by Wolpe when he used hypnotic procedures to facilitate the patient's experience of anxiety as he imagines himself approaching his phobic object or situation.

A therapeutic procedure based upon meditative practice was introduced in the 1920s by the German neuropsychiatrist J. H. Schultz. This is the technique of Autogenic Training, in which a state of quietude is induced by 'passive concentration' on bodily sensations such as 'heaviness in the arms' and warmth in the hands. The connection between this and Jacobsen's technique is readily apparent.

Exposure to Anxiety

Fear is strengthened by continued avoidance of the object feared, and encouragement to experience the fear as a step towards mastery is integral to most anxiety management techniques. Sigmund Freud recognized this in the context of his psychoanalytic therapy.

> 'One can hardly ever master a phobia if one waits till the patient lets the analyst influence him to give it up . . . [With agoraphobics] . . . one succeeds only when one can induce them . . . to go out in the street and struggle with their anxiety . . . it

is only when this has been achieved at the physician's demand that the associations and memories come into the patient's mind which enable the phobia to be resolved.'

Exposure to anxiety is fundamental to the success of anxiety management. Sometimes it is carried out in company of the therapist and sometimes the patient is encouraged to carry out his own exposure programme; sometimes it is introduced in a gradual manner as in Wolpe's procedure of systematic desensitization and sometimes encouragement is given for rapid exposure to anxiety at severe intensity. Sometimes the exposure is concentrated entirely towards the object that the patient presents as his phobia and sometimes, as in the technique of Implosion Therapy, the exposure is simply towards the concept of being anxious or nauseated or disgusted as he is encouraged to contemplate some unpleasant scenario.

The exposure may be towards some real psychotraumatic event. Abreaction was a technique devised to help the soldier overcome 'battle neurosis' in the First World War; under the influence of strong suggestion he was encouraged to visualize himself back in the terrifying ordeal which originally led to his state of anxiety, to reexperience so far as possible all the attendant emotion and thereby, it was hoped, to lose the fear through mastery of fear.

An interesting and sometimes surprisingly brief and effective exposure technique is Frankl's Paradoxical Intention; this is self-exposure to anxiety at maximum intensity and requires a sound grasp of the principle and strong motivation. The patient is instructed to expose himself to the feared situation and, instead of trying to control his anxiety, deliberately to intensify it. The therapist, of course, does nothing except 'sell' the technique to the patient but therein lies the skill: to explain it in such a way that it makes sense and the patient does not feel he is being mocked. An example will illustrate:

A young woman suffered from a disease which required repeated injections. She had a terror of hypodermic needles and of the sight of blood. The visits to the clinic were preceded by agonized misery and she invariably fainted as soon as she caught sight of the needle. The therapist gave her some hypodermic needles in their plastic coverings and she jumped as if she had been handed live snakes. She was encouraged to handle a needle in her own home many times a day, deliberately to induce as much anxiety as possible, to withdraw the needle from its case and finally to prick her finger and observe the spot of blood, over and over again. At her next visit to the clinic she did not faint and within a few weeks had lost her fear of the procedure.

Restructuring of Attitudes

Most people have deeply ingrained beliefs about themselves, their abilities and how other people must regard them. Frequently these beliefs are self-destructive, inhibiting the individual from engaging in activity which he might otherwise do with profit. Anxiety is fuelled by expectation that the dreaded event will occur and this maintains the anxiety; for instance, the young woman in the above case account believed she would feel anxious and faint and thereby increased her anxiety to the point where her expectation was inevitably fulfilled. The man with a sexual dysfunction of erectile impotence fears he will not maintain the erection long enough to satisfy his wife and so he forecasts the repetition of failure in each attempt at intercourse. The modification of these attitudes depends first upon their identification, to help the patient to become aware of the self-destructive attitudes and of how he reinforces them by what Meichenbaum calls his 'internal dialogue' with himself, what he says to himself as he approaches his problem area. Thus the agoraphobic patient, as she attempts to pass through her front door, may be engaged in the fearful thought that all the neighbours will be peering through their net-curtained windows at her, that she will inevitably show herself up to be stupid by falling down and losing control over her bowels and bladder.

Beck is one of the founding fathers of the cognitive approach to therapy. In a recent book written with colleagues *Anxiety Disorders and Phobias: A Cognitive Perspective*, they identify certain habits of thought which perpetuate anxiety: **exaggerating, catastrophizing, overgeneralizing** and **ignoring the positive**. In exaggerating the patient overemphasizes his existing defects. Catastrophizing is the tendency to predict total disaster in the anticipation of the attempt to engage upon any difficulty or danger. Overgeneralizing is the translation of a single failure to a law of failure in every aspect of life. An anxious person overlooks his successes but concentrates on his failure—this is 'ignoring the positive'. Beck's therapy induces the patient to become aware of his thoughts, to examine them for distortions of the above type, to substitute more balanced thoughts and to make plans to develop new and less destructive thought patterns.

A useful cognitive technique introduced by Meichenbaum is that of 'coping imagery'. The patient is asked repeatedly to visualize himself to be coping with stress, to be in control of the situation instead of becoming anxious and failing. This procedure of imaginative rehearsal is a useful technique whereby the patient may restructure his attitudes towards himself.

Self-Control

The traditional role of the healer is to assume the responsibility for bringing about the cure and this is the case whether the therapy is the prescription of medicines, achieving insight into distortion of mental processes or the laying on of hands. The role of the patient is to cooperate with the healer, to submit to his ministrations and to follow his instructions.

The concept of the patient as his own therapist has gathered pace in recent years and several strands of thought have contributed to it. First there is the evidence that many illnesses are not the operation of a blind and malevolent fate but are engendered by the patient himself; it is clear to many people that diseases resulting from overconsumption of food, intake of harmful substances and certain sexually transmitted diseases are the long-term risks of these indulgences. In the sphere of neurotic disorders cognitive psychologists are opening up the concept that faulty attitudes and patterns of self-destructive thinking are at the root of much of the trouble and that once this is pointed out then the patient must take responsibility for change, for without motivation to change and effort to do so all psychotherapeutic endeavours will fail. However, this apparently obvious conclusion was largely overlooked until a generation of North American psychologists including Meichenbaum, Bandura and Kanfer began to publish their thoughts. Kanfer has reinterpreted the role of the therapist as a consultant who negotiates with a client how to go about change and to what end. The whole prior emphasis of psychotherapy, behavioural as well as explorative varieties, is then turned round so that attention is no longer focused upon past experience but repertoires for dealing with the future are explored and skills developed to deal with problems which might arise. Change will be more successful and more likely to endure when the patient perceives his own responsibility for distress, rather than attributing it to someone or something else, and then accepts a major responsibility for change.

Important elements in the process of self-management are those of self-monitoring and the establishment of goals through clearly understood mechanisms laid down as a contract between the patient and the therapist; such a contract may, for example in an obese person, involve studying throughout the lunch hour instead of going to the college canteen. Self-monitoring may be aided by a 'diary' or other device in which the patient notes the occurrence of distress symptoms and the circumstances in which they appeared.

An Anxiety Management Technique

An example will now be presented of a technique which incorporates the foregoing principles of anxiety management. The technique is called Anxiety Control Training (ACT) and is more fully described by one of us in the text *Clinical Neurosis* (Snaith, 1981). It is readily conducted by any health professional with little prior training and it is suitable for health service practice since it requires little of the therapist's time; the patient conducts his own treatment under direction from the therapist over a series of about eight weekly 15-minute sessions. It can be adapted for group treatment.

Preparation for Treatment

Having been thought to be suitable for help by ACT, the patient is given a pamphlet (see Appendix 7.1) describing the method. He is asked to read it, think about it, perhaps discuss it with a relative and then to decide whether he wishes to be instructed in the ACT programme. The booklet makes it clear that a successful outcome depends upon regular homework practice of a technique of self-control demonstrated by the therapist; two 10-minute sessions a day must be set aside for the therapy and attendance at the weekly sessions must be regular. Self-discipline is the key to success. Having decided to accept ACT the patient is informed that he will be shown how to enter a state of trance, and that this state is a natural one which will not be imposed upon him and which he will be able, with practice, to conduct for himself. The purpose of the trance is to learn to induce a state of calm. After a few sessions, when a degree of proficiency has been obtained, he will be shown how to let an anxious feeling replace the calm state during the sessions in order to learn the skill of controlling the anxiety. After a few weeks of homework practice he will find that he can automatically control anxiety in real-life situations by thinking of his coping phrase 'Calm, control'; with continued practice his self-confidence will increase and with that the anxiety and phobias will fade away.

The value of the trance in heightening suggestibility and thus making suggested and self-suggested scenes feel real is discussed.

Trance Induction

The difference between the technique and conventional hypnosis is discussed. In hypnosis trance is induced by the hypnotist, but in ACT the therapist merely provides the optimum conditions for the facilitation of trance induction by the patient himself. A chair with head and arm rests is preferable and ideally one which is adjustable so that the patient may sit upright or lie back in the position which he finds to be most comfortable; the instruction to find the comfortable position underlines the theme of self rather than therapist control of the session. Having found the comfortable position, the patient is instructed to fixate his gaze on some point opposite as an aid to concentration; he is informed that, as the session proceeds, he may let his eyes close but there is no instruction that he *must* close his eyes and some patients prefer to conduct the sessions with their eyes open throughout. The instruction is then given to concentrate on the therapist's words and, through concentration, to allow relaxation and the other effects to come about. The therapist then speaks in a quiet, but of course audible, voice and as the session proceeds leaves longer pauses between phrases, so allowing the patient to take control.

There is no standard formula of words but the induction should last about five to ten minutes; longer periods of attention are difficult to sustain. However, the therapist should first draw attention to somatic sensations and then to mental imagery, allowing the patient to choose the latter for himself. The following is an example of an induction procedure:

> 'Now resting comfortably back . . . just letting your gaze rest upon the point you have chosen and listening to my voice . . . as the relaxation continues your eyes may wish to close in order to enjoy deeper calm in which case they will . . . think first about your hands [the therapist observes the position of the hands in order not to make contradictory statements]. Just thinking of the position of your hands . . . the slight contact or pressure of the palms of your hands, the tips of your fingers on the chair rest . . . now the warmth or the coolness, that is the temperature of the skin of your hands . . . whether they are warm or cool . . . and any other feelings you may notice, perhaps slight tingling feelings in your hands . . . and

now your arms, the position of your arms . . . your shoulders resting against the back of the chair . . . becoming aware of any tension . . . or tightness in the muscles of your arms, round your shoulders and neck . . . tension or tightness now becoming replaced by relaxation so your arms now begin to feel limp and relaxed . . . just letting relaxation come, that's good . . . arms limp and relaxed . . . and just letting controlled relaxation begin to come all through your body, not resisting it, just inviting this controlled relaxation . . . now your feet and legs, just like with your hands and arms, first your feet and all the feelings you notice . . . the position of your feet, warmth or coolness, that is the temperature of the skin of your feet . . . whether they are warm or cool . . . and other feelings, tingling feelings and so on . . . the position of your legs, the pressure of the back of your legs against the chair rest . . . and becoming aware of tightness in your legs — replaced by relaxation . . . like your arms, limp and relaxed . . . now the muscles of your stomach and chest . . . tension, knotted up tension feelings replaced by relaxation — . . . sinking back deeper into the chair . . . deeper with the relaxation . . . not resisting but inviting controlled relaxation . . . now your face muscles, around your forehead and eyes, frowning tension replaced by smooth relaxation . . . forehead muscles smooth and relaxed — deeper [If eyes not closed by this stage the therapist may give permission to close the eyes] . . . many people like to let their eyes close at this stage, in order to enjoy deeper relaxation, but you do what you like, eyes open or closed, whichever is comfortable . . . and the muscles of your jaws, clenching teeth tension . . . replaced by relaxation . . . that's good, a deep controlled, calm relaxation all through you and taking time to enjoy this control . . . your control over tension . . . now let come into your mind's eye a picture, a calm picture . . . most people choose a picture of somewhere they know or flowers but you choose just what you want . . . your picture . . . and through the picture deeper still into controlled calm relaxation . . . as you go on with your homework practice you will find it easier to bring in this deep controlled calm feeling . . . now I'm going to stop talking altogether and you may continue with your calm controlled relaxation for a little longer . . . and then, in your own time and when it suits you, bring the session to an end . . . in your own time. . . .'

It will be noted that, in accord with the principle of trance induction, statements are phrased in the passive voice: 'your arms become relaxed . . . a picture comes to your mind . . .', and so forth. After the session the patient is then asked to give an account of his experience; especially at the first session clear imagery may be absent, but a statement of some type of bodily sensation is useful in instruction for home practice and this is the reason for directing attention to various parts of the body during the induction. The patient is warned that self-induction of the trance is more difficult than the therapist-guided session and is best carried out by the selection of no more than two phrases which are used to concentrate thought and fend off distracting thoughts that repeatedly enter the mind. If there has been a definite somatic sensation the words may be used for induction of the same sensation in the home practice; the self-induction of the sensation is a 'success experience' which reinforces interest and application to the programme.

Anxiety Induction

At about the third session, when progress is being made with trance induction, anxiety is introduced. The therapist explains that, once the patient is in the trance and experiencing his calm scene, the suggestion will be given that some scene inducing a slight feeling of discomfort will replace the calm scene and that the purpose is to practise control over anxiety. The patient should be told that it does not matter what anxiety-inducing situation he brings to mind since anxiety control training teaches a general mastery over anxiety rather than focusing on specific phobias. However, it is advisable to commence with a situation producing only slight discomfort and work towards the more distressing situations as confidence increases. The trance is then induced in the usual way and the therapist proceeds along the following lines:

'You are now in your calm scene, in full control over anxiety but shortly you will leave the calm scene and go over to a situation which makes you feel a little uncomfortable. When this happens your hand, the one I am touching, will twitch or move a little and I shall then know you are experiencing discomfort. [At this point the therapist actually touches one of the patient's hands leaving no doubt as to how anxiety will be signalled.] Don't think any more about your hand, it will just move automatically when you feel anxious. Now, you are beginning to move away from the calm scene to your uncomfortable situation, just take your time, at your own pace . . . [The therapist becomes silent and watches the patient closely; sometimes the hand movement is so slight that it would be missed without close inspection and sometimes the hand does not move but there is other evidence of distress such as a frowning expression, increased respiration rate or general fidgeting movements. As soon as the therapist observes a signal of discomfort he continues . . .] You are now feeling a little uncomfortable but you can control that feeling by just letting the words CALM, CONTROL go through your mind . . . that's right, the words CALM, CONTROL controlling anxiety . . . and as you continue with this practice on your own at home you will find that you have more and more confidence in your ability to control anxiety in everyday life by just thinking the words CALM, CONTROL whenever you begin to feel anxious.'

Usually the patient does not need to be directed to specific anxiety-arousing situations; he directs himself towards the situations which trouble him most. Once anxiety has been induced and successfully controlled in the therapy sessions the patient is instructed to start to introduce anxiety into the homework sessions. At first he may be a little reluctant to do this or reports that his attempts are not successful, which generally signifies that he has not yet developed the confidence in self-control over anxiety that will come with a further few sessions with the therapist. He may also be attempting to envisage situations which cause too much anxiety, in which case he should be advised to choose scenes causing less distress until his confidence to tackle the more severe ones increases.

Restructuring of Attitudes

An important part of the programme is the management to resume positive self-statements in place of self-defeating predictions of failure and inability to exert mastery over anxiety. The therapist should spend a few minutes at each session enquiring about difficulties experienced in home practice and pointing out that, in the early stages, it is the common experience to have some difficulty in concentration. Motivation must be reinforced and at the same time there should not be expectation of rapid progress. Mastery over anxiety advances by small steps and it is helpful to point out that pressure to encounter anxiety-provoking situations in real life should be resisted; most people find that, with regular application to the programme, they almost unthinkingly broaden their sphere of activity.

The therapist should take note of any 'success experiences' mentioned by the patient and, however small these may be, should 'reward' with interest and further encouragement. It is important for the patient to know that the therapist considers him to be 'on course' and is not discouraged that he is not making faster progress. At a late stage in therapy the patient may benefit from a more direct encouragement to enter anxiety-provoking situations.

The pervading theme of ACT is that self-mastery can occur if the patient wills it and is prepared to work towards that goal.

Further Considerations

Anxiety control training may be successful in helping the patient to cope with unalterable situations of personal adversity where control of anxiety will not change the situations but will enable the patient to feel more confident and therefore to cope better with adversity, whether this be difficulties in personal relationships, severe illness or even approaching death. It will also be apparent that ACT is an exercise in the development of self-control in a wider sense than just anxiety control. As such, it may be used in impulse control disorders such as impulsive eating, drinking or some types of offensive behaviour such as exhibitionism. Similar meditative techniques have been used in the successful treatment of some tension-based physical disorders such as hypertension.

The method is, of course, not always successful; the commonest cause for failure is lack of motivation for change and compliance with the requirements of attendance and home practice. Relatives interfere with application to the method and progress for they may sometimes covertly wish to maintain the patient in the sick or dependent role. It is always useful to discuss the programme with the nearest relative as well as the patient before commencement.

> A nine-year-old girl was referred for a simple phobia of dogs. She was extremely keen to overcome the fear and accepted the demands of the programme. However, her progress was poor; her mother had remarried and actually forbade the child to see her father which caused her much distress. The mother was a curiously selfish and unfeeling woman who appeared to bolster her own poor self-esteem by having a daughter who was unhappy. It was not until these family dynamics were explored and discussed that therapy could proceed.

The biogenic depressive state of anhedonia frequently accompanies clinical anxiety states and the nature of this relationship was discussed in Chapter 3. It is important that even mild degrees of the disorder should be detected and appropriately treated before proceeding with ACT. In this form of depressive state motivation is impeded and the self-rewarding responses, so important to progress with ACT, are diminished. As already pointed out, psychological treatments in the presence of anhedonic depression are not likely to succeed and exhortation to engage in them only produces another failure experience, leading the patient a step nearer to despair. The use of the HAD Scale (Chapter 6) to monitor treatment is a useful aid to the detection of depressive anhedonia; the chart shown in Figure 7.1 records a case where depression inhibited progress with ACT, but, once this was successfully treated with imipramine, the anxiety state responded to resumption of the psychotherapeutic programme.

FURTHER READING

Bloch, Sidney. *What is Psychotherapy?* Oxford; Oxford University Press, 1982.
Kovel, Joel. *A Complete Guide To Therapy.* Harmondsworth: Penguin, 1978.

Appendix 7.1:

Anxiety Control Training

The following text and the Anxiety Scale in Appendix 6.1 may be used to form an explanatory pamphlet which can be given to a patient prior to commencing the therapy. Reproduction of this text is free of charge subject to acknowledgement of the source on all such reproductions.

Anxiety is a normal emotion. In situations of danger we feel anxious and this prompts us to remove ourselves from the dangerous situation. However, anxiety can get out of control and many people feel very anxious in situations which are really not dangerous or else the extent of the danger becomes exaggerated. A list of situations in which many people experience unnecessary anxiety is printed at the end of this pamphlet and you may find it helpful to look at the list and see whether any apply to you.

Anxiety is a very uncomfortable experience. There is a feeling of fear, certain bodily sensations such as the heart beating fast, being unable to breathe in enough air, flushing of the skin, sweating, dry mouth and, in persistent anxiety, muscle pains. Overbreathing frequently occurs and this leads to other unpleasant bodily sensations such as dizziness, tingling in the fingers and muscle spasms. There is often an overpowering urge to leave the situation where these sensations occur. Leaving the situation may bring about relief but the trouble then is that a vicious circle soon builds up, with increasing fear of the situation until sometimes it is quite impossible to enter that situation at all. At other times the anxiety may not occur in particular situations but there is a persistent feeling of anxiety which causes the person to feel restless, jumpy, fearful that something awful is about to occur although exactly what is not known, and fearful thoughts or worries that serve no useful purpose go on and on, sometimes preventing sleep. This persistent anxiety may suddenly reach a severe degree, often for no reason the person can understand, and this alarming experience is called a panic attack.

The result of all this unnecessary anxiety is that the sufferer often restricts his lifestyle. He, or she, may feel very foolish that he feels anxious when other people apparently do not, he may start to rely on sedative drugs which after a while stop helping or he may use alcoholic drinks to give him false courage. The state of demoralization sets in when a person feels that he cannot do anything to control anxiety, that he is helpless in the face of it.

This programme of self-help, called Anxiety Control Training, is designed to enable the person to learn mastery over anxiety. It will only work if the person wishes to learn the skill of controlling anxiety and it has to be worked at steadily and regularly over several weeks. There is no short cut. It is therefore very important that you should make up your mind whether you want to apply yourself to learning anxiety control since it is only through your own efforts that improvement will occur. If you do decide you want to do it let your therapist know and he, or she, will show you how to get started.

The therapist will show you a method of achieving a state of calm relaxation simply by concentrating your mind on words that he speaks; some therapists use tape-recorded words. Whichever method is used, through concentration on the words, which are concerned with relaxation replacing tension throughout your body and a calm thought or picture coming to your mind's eye, you will after a session or two be able to experience a feeling of calm. Then you practise doing this for yourself, quite regularly, preferably twice but at least once a day. Sessions should not be long — just 10 minutes. You will need to be in a room on your own to carry out a session, and it is difficult to do if you are very tired, so avoid such times.

To do your own session you concentrate on certain words or thoughts which your therapist will have discussed with you. It is hard to do this at first because your thoughts keep wandering but with practice and further sessions with the therapist you will learn how to 'clear your mind' and induce for yourself a state of calmness. You may at first think it would be easier to have a tape recording to carry out your homework sessions, but it is better to learn to rely on yourself rather than some external device. When you become more practised you will then know that you can induce your calm state at any time which suits you.

After you have had a few sessions the therapist will show you how to let anxious feelings replace calm feelings while you are carrying out a session. The point of that is so that you may find out a simple method of controlling the anxiety, perhaps through the thought of key words such as CALM, CONTROL. You will then be asked to practise doing that in your homework and, after a while, you will find that in 'real life' situations, when you feel unnecessary anxiety building up, you will be able to exert some degree of control over it. With further practice your mastery over anxiety improves steadily and at this stage you will find yourself coping with situations which previously you dreaded or which were impossible for you. The list of situations comprises the Focused Anxiety Schedule (page 79).

The really good thing about Anxiety Control Training is that *you* do it, not the therapist or someone else doing it to you. And once you have acquired the skill of controlling anxiety, learned where the 'panic button' is, then it is yours for life. You don't need to keep going for 'top-ups' or have to continue to rely on your therapist being around.

Anxiety Control Training is really very simple, and a pleasant way of learning to help yourself. But remember: it won't help unless you have really made up your mind that you are going to work at it.

Appendix:

Self-Help Organizations in the United Kingdom

Open Door Association

> Secretary: Mrs Mona Woodford, MBE
> 447 Pensby Road
> Heswall
> Wirral
> Cheshire
> L61 9PQ

An organization which attempts to encourage people to use self-help towards recovery from anxiety states, stress and agoraphobia. Cassettes and book available. Supply stamped addressed envelope when requesting information.

Action on Phobias

> Contact person: Shandy Mathias
> 8 The Avenue
> Eastbourne
> East Sussex
> BN21 3YA

To help those suffering from phobia or general anxiety difficulties to overcome their fears and live without the restrictions and distress they create.

The organization establishes local self-help groups and a telephone link line. It also provides cassette training programmes. Always enclose stamped addressed envelope.

Phobic Action

> Greater London House
> 547/551 High Road
> Leytonstone
> London E11 4PR
>
> Office: 01-558 3463
>
> Helpline: 01-558 6012

Phobic action is a Registered National Charity No 296746 which provides support, advice and assistance to local self-help groups. Services provided include a national help-line telephone, home visiting, branch support and training, advice packs, local meetings and a regular newsletter. National advisers include the Rt Hon Lord Ennals, Dr John Horder and Professor Isaac Marks.
Membership £5.00 a year.

Tranx

> National Tranquillizer Advice Centre
> 25a Masons Avenue
> Wealdstone
> Harrow
> Middlesex
> HA3 5AH
>
> 01-863 9716/01-427 2827 (24 hours answering service)
>
> (Client line) 01-427 2065

Information and advice for those who have problems with tranquillizers. Offers information to the medical profession, para-professionals, welfare and personnel officers in industry and commerce and all community workers.
Creates greater awareness in the community of the consequences of long-term minor tranquillizer/sleeping pill use.
Issues a quarterly newsletter available at an annual subscription fee.

Index